PCOS DIET COOKBOOK FOR BEGINNERS

A Comprehensive Recipe Guide for Hormone-Balanced Eating

BY

Hector Wiggins

Table of Contents

INTRODUCTION

In the quiet corners of bustling kitchens, amidst the sizzle of sauté pans and the gentle hum of blenders, there exists a narrative of resilience, empowerment, and transformation. It's a narrative woven into the fabric of every recipe, every ingredient meticulously selected, and every meal shared with intention. **Welcome to "Pcos Diet Cookbook - A Journey Through PCOS,"** where the art of culinary alchemy meets the science of nourishment, offering a beacon of hope and healing to those navigating the labyrinthine landscape of Polycystic Ovary Syndrome (PCOS).

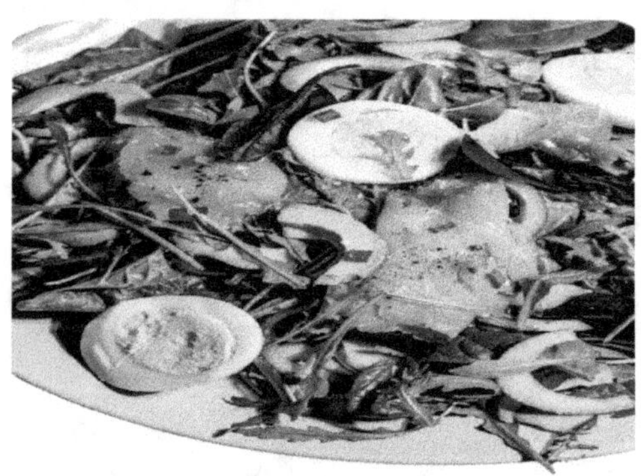

Our story begins not with medical jargon or clinical diagnoses, but with a journey of self-discovery and unwavering determination. Picture, if you will, a young woman standing at the crossroads of uncertainty, her path obscured by the shadows of unanswered questions and unspoken fears. **Her name is Emma, and like millions of women around the world, she finds herself grappling with the enigmatic complexities of PCOS.**

For Emma, PCOS was more than just a diagnosis; it was a formidable adversary that threatened to overshadow her dreams of health, happiness, and fulfillment. From the insidious weight gain and hormonal imbalances to the harrowing battle with infertility, each day seemed to herald a new trial, a new tribulation. Yet, amidst the chaos and confusion, Emma refused to surrender to despair. Instead, she embarked on a quest for knowledge, seeking solace in the wisdom of ancient traditions and the cutting-edge insights of modern science.

It was through this journey of self-empowerment that Emma discovered the transformative power of food - not merely as sustenance for the body, but as medicine for the soul. Guided by the gentle whispers of intuition and the unwavering support of her community, she embarked on a culinary odyssey, exploring the rich tapestry of flavors, textures, and aromas that the world had to offer.

With each recipe she crafted, Emma found herself reclaiming a sense of agency, a sense of control over her own well-being. Gone were the days of deprivation and despair; in their place blossomed a newfound sense of vitality, radiance, and joy. Through trial and error, experimentation and adaptation, she began to unravel the intricate dance of hormones and nutrients, crafting meals that not only nourished her body but nourished her spirit as well.

And so, "Pcos Diet Cookbook - A Journey Through PCOS" was born - not as a mere collection of recipes, but as a testament to the indomitable power of the human spirit. Within these pages, you will find a treasure trove of culinary delights, each one carefully curated to support hormonal balance, promote metabolic health, and ignite the flames of vitality within.

But beyond the realm of food lies a deeper truth - a truth that transcends the boundaries of diet and disease. It is the truth that within each and every one of us resides the innate capacity for healing, for growth, for transformation.

It is the truth that no matter how daunting the journey may seem, we are never truly alone; for in the kitchen of life, we are all connected by the universal language of love, nourishment, and wellness.

So join us, dear reader, as we embark on a journey of healing, of hope, of wholeness. Let us gather around the communal table of abundance, breaking bread and breaking barriers, one delicious bite at a time. For in the sacred act of nourishing ourselves, we discover the infinite potential that lies dormant within - the potential to thrive, to flourish, to live our lives with boundless vitality and grace.

Welcome to "Pcos Diet Cookbook - A Journey Through PCOS." May this cookbook be a guiding light on your path to wellness, a reminder that within every challenge lies the seeds of opportunity, and within every meal lies the promise of healing.

Understanding PCOS and its dietary implications

Millions of women worldwide suffer from the complex endocrine condition known as polycystic ovarian syndrome (PCOS). PCOS, which is characterized by ovarian cysts, hormonal imbalances, and metabolic disturbances, poses a wide range of difficulties that go well beyond reproductive health. Although the precise etiology of PCOS is still unknown, scientists think it is a complex disorder influenced by a person's genetics, insulin resistance, and lifestyle choices.

One of the key hallmarks of PCOS is insulin resistance, a condition in which the body's cells become less responsive to the effects of insulin, leading to elevated blood sugar levels and increased insulin production by the pancreas. Insulin resistance is closely linked to obesity and plays a central role in the pathophysiology of PCOS, contributing to the development of metabolic abnormalities such as type 2 diabetes, dyslipidemia, and cardiovascular disease.

The hormonal imbalances associated with PCOS, including elevated levels of androgens (male hormones) such as testosterone, can disrupt the normal function of the menstrual cycle and contribute to symptoms such as irregular periods, acne, hirsutism (excessive hair growth), and hair loss. Additionally, these hormonal fluctuations can impact metabolism, appetite regulation, and energy expenditure, making weight management particularly challenging for women with PCOS.

Given the intricate interplay between hormones, metabolism, and dietary factors in PCOS, adopting a tailored approach to nutrition is essential for managing symptoms and promoting overall health and well-being. While there is no one-size-fits-all diet for PCOS, several dietary strategies have shown promise in improving insulin sensitivity, reducing androgen levels, and supporting hormonal balance.

One such approach is the low glycemic index (GI) diet, which emphasizes foods that have a minimal impact on blood sugar levels. By choosing carbohydrates that are digested and absorbed more slowly, such as whole grains, legumes, fruits, and vegetables, individuals with PCOS can help stabilize blood sugar levels, reduce insulin resistance, and improve metabolic health.

In addition to focusing on low GI carbohydrates, a balanced PCOS diet should include adequate protein and healthy fats to promote satiety, stabilize blood sugar levels, and support hormone production. Lean sources of protein, such as poultry, fish, tofu, and legumes, provide essential amino acids for tissue repair and muscle synthesis, while healthy fats from sources such as avocados, nuts, seeds, and olive oil help reduce inflammation and support hormone synthesis.

Furthermore, incorporating plenty of fiber-rich foods into the diet, such as fruits, vegetables, whole grains, and legumes, can aid in digestion, promote feelings of fullness, and regulate blood sugar levels. Fiber also plays a crucial role in gut health, promoting the growth of beneficial bacteria and reducing the risk of insulin resistance and metabolic dysfunction.

In contrast, certain dietary factors may exacerbate symptoms of PCOS and should be limited or avoided altogether. These include highly processed foods, sugary snacks and beverages, refined carbohydrates, and trans fats, which can contribute to insulin resistance, inflammation, and weight gain. Additionally, dairy products and foods high in saturated fats may exacerbate hormonal imbalances in some women with PCOS and may be best consumed in moderation or replaced with healthier alternatives.

Let's sum up by saying that knowing the dietary consequences of PCOS is crucial for controlling symptoms, enhancing metabolic health, and fostering general wellbeing. Women with PCOS can empower themselves to take charge of their health, enhance their quality of life, and thrive despite the obstacles presented by this complex condition by implementing a balanced and customized approach to nutrition. Collaborating closely with medical specialists, such as endocrinologists and registered dietitians, can offer priceless support and direction in navigating the PCOS dietary maze and attaining long-term health and wellness.

How this cookbook can help manage PCOS symptoms through diet

Navigating the complexities of Polycystic Ovary Syndrome (PCOS) can feel like traversing a labyrinth with no clear path forward. From hormonal imbalances to metabolic disturbances, the symptoms of PCOS can have far-reaching effects on physical, emotional, and psychological well-being. However, amidst the challenges lie opportunities for empowerment, and one of the most potent tools in the arsenal against PCOS is a carefully crafted diet.

This cookbook is more than just a collection of recipes; it is a roadmap to reclaiming control over your health and flourishing in spite of PCOS. Here's how this cookbook can help you manage PCOS symptoms through diet:

1. **Tailored Nutritional Guidance**: Unlike generic diet plans, this cookbook is specifically designed to address the unique dietary needs and challenges faced by individuals with PCOS. Each recipe is thoughtfully curated to support hormonal balance, stabilize blood sugar levels, and promote metabolic health, offering a roadmap to optimal nutrition tailored to your condition.

2. **Focus on Whole, Nutrient-Dense Foods**: The recipes featured in this cookbook prioritize whole, nutrient-dense ingredients that nourish the body from the inside out. From vibrant fruits and vegetables to lean proteins and healthy fats, each recipe is carefully crafted to provide the essential vitamins, minerals, and antioxidants needed to support overall health and well-being.

3. **Emphasis on Low Glycemic Index Foods**: Given the central role of insulin resistance in PCOS, this cookbook places a strong emphasis on incorporating low glycemic index (GI) foods into your diet. By choosing carbohydrates that are digested and absorbed more slowly, you can help stabilize blood sugar levels, reduce insulin resistance, and improve metabolic health.

4. **Balanced Macronutrient Ratios**: Achieving a balanced macronutrient ratio is crucial for managing PCOS symptoms, and this cookbook provides recipes that are rich in protein, healthy fats, and complex carbohydrates. By prioritizing these macronutrients, you can support hormone production, promote satiety, and maintain stable energy levels throughout the day.

5. **Variety and Flavor:** Eating healthily doesn't have to be boring, and this cookbook proves that delicious, flavorful meals can also be nourishing and supportive of PCOS management. From hearty breakfasts to satisfying dinners and indulgent desserts, there's a diverse array of recipes to suit every taste and preference, ensuring that you never feel deprived or restricted in your culinary choices.

6. **Practical Tips and Strategies**: In addition to mouthwatering recipes, this cookbook also provides practical tips and strategies for meal planning, grocery shopping, and batch cooking. These resources empower you to take charge of your nutrition and make informed choices that support your PCOS management goals.

7. **Holistic Approach to Wellness**: Managing PCOS goes beyond just diet; it encompasses all aspects of health and well-being. That's why this cookbook takes a holistic approach, addressing lifestyle factors such as exercise, stress management, and sleep hygiene alongside dietary considerations. By embracing a comprehensive approach to wellness, you can optimize your chances of success in managing PCOS symptoms and living your best life.

In summary, this cookbook is a guide to regaining your health, energy, and sense of agency despite PCOS, not just a list of recipes. With its focus on complete, nutrient-dense foods, balanced macronutrient ratios, and helpful success advice, this cookbook gives you the knowledge and resources you need to thrive in spite of PCOS's obstacles. Now get your hands dirty, sharpen your knives, and set out on a mouthwatering culinary exploration that will fill you up, calm your spirit, and give you the tools you need to take charge of your health one delicious bite at a time.

CHAPTER ONE

PCOS Basics

Polycystic Ovary Syndrome (PCOS) stands as one of the most prevalent endocrine disorders affecting women of reproductive age worldwide. Despite its prevalence, PCOS remains a complex and multifaceted condition, often shrouded in misconceptions and misunderstanding. Delving into the PCOS basics illuminates the intricate web of symptoms, diagnostic criteria, and underlying mechanisms that define this syndrome.

1. Definition and Prevalence:

PCOS is characterized by a combination of hormonal imbalances, ovarian dysfunction, and metabolic disturbances. While the exact cause of PCOS remains elusive, genetic predisposition, insulin resistance, and environmental factors are believed to play significant roles in its development. PCOS affects approximately 5-10% of women of reproductive age, making it one of the most common endocrine disorders worldwide.

2. **Diagnostic Criteria:**

The diagnosis of PCOS is typically based on a combination of clinical, biochemical, and imaging criteria. The Rotterdam criteria, established by the European Society for Human Reproduction and Embryology (ESHRE) and the American Society for Reproductive Medicine (ASRM), include the presence of two out of three of the following features: irregular or absent menstrual cycles (oligomenorrhea or amenorrhea), clinical or biochemical signs of hyperandrogenism (such as hirsutism, acne, or elevated testosterone levels), and polycystic ovaries visualized on ultrasound.

3. **Hormonal Imbalances:**

PCOS is characterized by disruptions in the normal balance of reproductive hormones, including elevated levels of androgens (male hormones) such as testosterone, luteinizing hormone (LH), and insulin-like growth factor 1 (IGF-1). These hormonal imbalances can disrupt the normal function of the menstrual cycle, leading to irregular periods, anovulation (lack of ovulation), and infertility.

4. Ovarian Dysfunction:

One of the defining features of PCOS is the presence of ovarian cysts, which are small fluid-filled sacs that develop within the ovaries. These cysts result from the abnormal maturation of ovarian follicles and contribute to the characteristic appearance of "polycystic" ovaries on ultrasound. While ovarian cysts are a common feature of PCOS, not all women with PCOS will have visible cysts, and their absence does not rule out the diagnosis.

5. Metabolic Disturbances:

Insulin resistance and obesity are common comorbidities in women with PCOS and are thought to exacerbate the hormonal and reproductive abnormalities associated with the condition. Insulin resistance occurs when the body's cells become less responsive to the effects of insulin, leading to elevated blood sugar levels and increased insulin production by the pancreas. This metabolic dysfunction can contribute to weight gain, dyslipidemia, and an increased risk of type 2 diabetes and cardiovascular disease in women with PCOS.

6. **Impact on Reproductive Health:**
PCOS can have significant implications for reproductive health, including infertility, miscarriage, and pregnancy complications such as gestational diabetes and pre-eclampsia. The hormonal imbalances and ovulatory dysfunction characteristic of PCOS can make it challenging for women to conceive naturally, necessitating fertility treatments such as ovulation induction or assisted reproductive technologies (ART) in some cases.

7. **Psychological and Emotional Effects:**
Beyond its physical manifestations, PCOS can also take a toll on psychological and emotional well-being, contributing to symptoms such as depression, anxiety, and poor self-esteem. The hormonal fluctuations, menstrual irregularities, and body image concerns associated with PCOS can exacerbate existing mental health issues and significantly impact quality of life.

What is PCOS?

Polycystic ovary syndrome (PCOS) is a hormonal
disorder that affects people of reproductive age,
particularly women. It's characterized by a
combination of symptoms that can vary from person
to person. The exact cause of PCOS is unknown,
but it's believed to involve a combination of genetic
and environmental factors.

One of the key features of PCOS is irregular
menstrual periods. This can manifest as infrequent
periods, prolonged periods, or unpredictable
bleeding. Another hallmark of PCOS is an excess of
androgens, which are male hormones that females
also produce in smaller amounts. This hormonal
imbalance can lead to symptoms such as acne,
excessive facial and body hair (hirsutism), and
male-pattern baldness.

Furthermore, PCOS often involves the presence of multiple cysts on the ovaries. These cysts are small fluid-filled sacs and are typically harmless, but their presence contributes to the syndrome's name. However, not all people with PCOS will have cysts on their ovaries, and not all ovarian cysts indicate PCOS.

PCOS can also affect fertility. Irregular ovulation or lack of ovulation can make it more difficult for women with PCOS to conceive. Additionally, PCOS is associated with an increased risk of other health issues, including insulin resistance, type 2 diabetes, high cholesterol, high blood pressure, and sleep apnea. There may also be an increased risk of developing endometrial cancer due to irregular menstrual cycles and prolonged exposure to estrogen without progesterone.

Diagnosing PCOS involves evaluating a person's medical history, symptoms, and physical examination, as well as performing various tests, such as blood tests to measure hormone levels, ultrasound imaging of the ovaries to look for cysts, and sometimes other tests to assess metabolic health.

The goals of PCOS treatment are to control symptoms and lower the chance of complications. To control weight and enhance insulin sensitivity, this may entail dietary and exercise modifications. In addition, doctors may prescribe medication to treat other symptoms, lower testosterone levels, enhance fertility, or control menstrual cycles. Surgery might be suggested in some circumstances to treat infertility or remove ovarian cysts. In general, PCOS sufferers can live healthier lives with early diagnosis and proper care.

Causes and symptoms of PCOS

Polycystic Ovary Syndrome (PCOS) is a multifaceted endocrine disorder characterized by hormonal imbalances, ovarian dysfunction, and metabolic disturbances. While the exact cause of PCOS remains elusive, researchers believe it to be a combination of genetic, environmental, and lifestyle factors. Understanding the interplay between these factors is crucial for unraveling the complexities of PCOS and developing effective treatment strategies.

Causes of PCOS:

Genetic Predisposition: There appears to be a genetic component to PCOS, as individuals with a family history of the condition are at increased risk of developing it themselves. Specific genes implicated in PCOS include those involved in hormone regulation, insulin sensitivity, and ovarian function.

Hormonal Imbalances: PCOS is characterized by elevated levels of androgens (male hormones) such as testosterone, as well as disruptions in other hormones such as insulin, luteinizing hormone (LH), and follicle-stimulating hormone (FSH). These hormonal imbalances contribute to the symptoms and manifestations of PCOS, including irregular menstrual cycles, ovarian cysts, and hirsutism.

Insulin Resistance: Insulin resistance is a common feature of PCOS, occurring in approximately 70-80% of affected individuals. Insulin resistance occurs when the body's cells become less responsive to the effects of insulin, leading to elevated blood sugar levels and increased insulin production by the pancreas. This metabolic dysfunction is thought to exacerbate the hormonal imbalances and ovarian dysfunction characteristic of PCOS.

Environmental and Lifestyle Factors:
Environmental factors such as exposure to
endocrine-disrupting chemicals (EDCs) and
lifestyle factors such as diet, exercise, and stress
may also contribute to the development and
progression of PCOS. High levels of stress, poor
dietary habits, and sedentary lifestyles can
exacerbate insulin resistance and hormonal
imbalances, further complicating the management
of PCOS.

Symptoms of PCOS:

Menstrual Irregularities: Irregular menstrual
cycles, including oligomenorrhea (infrequent
periods) or amenorrhea (absence of periods), are
common in individuals with PCOS due to ovulatory
dysfunction.

Ovarian Dysfunction: PCOS is characterized by
the presence of multiple small follicular cysts
within the ovaries, which can be visualized on
ultrasound imaging. These cysts result from
abnormal follicular development and contribute to
the characteristic appearance of "polycystic"
ovaries.

Hyperandrogenism: Elevated levels of androgens, such as testosterone, can lead to symptoms of hyperandrogenism, including hirsutism (excessive hair growth), acne, male-pattern baldness, and acanthosis nigricans (darkening of the skin in body creases).

Metabolic Disturbances: Insulin resistance and obesity are common comorbidities in individuals with PCOS and can lead to metabolic disturbances such as weight gain, abdominal obesity, dyslipidemia, and an increased risk of type 2 diabetes and cardiovascular disease.

Reproductive Health Implications: PCOS can have significant implications for reproductive health, including infertility, miscarriage, and pregnancy complications such as gestational diabetes and pre-eclampsia. The combination of hormonal imbalances and ovulatory dysfunction can make it challenging for individuals with PCOS to conceive naturally, necessitating fertility treatments such as ovulation induction or assisted reproductive technologies (ART).

In conclusion, PCOS is a complex and heterogeneous condition with a multitude of underlying causes and a diverse array of symptoms. By understanding the genetic, hormonal, environmental, and lifestyle factors that contribute to PCOS, healthcare providers can develop personalized treatment plans that address the unique needs and challenges of each individual with PCOS. Early detection, intervention, and comprehensive management are crucial in mitigating the long-term health implications of PCOS and improving the quality of life for affected individuals.

How PCOS affects diet and nutrition

Polycystic Ovary Syndrome (PCOS) is a complex endocrine disorder that can have profound effects on diet, nutrition, and overall metabolic health. Understanding how PCOS impacts diet and nutrition is crucial for individuals with the condition and healthcare professionals alike, as dietary interventions play a significant role in managing PCOS symptoms and improving long-term health outcomes.

1. Insulin Resistance and Blood Sugar Management:

One of the key features of PCOS is insulin resistance, a condition in which the body's cells become less responsive to the effects of insulin. Insulin resistance leads to elevated blood sugar levels and increased insulin production by the pancreas. As a result, individuals with PCOS may experience difficulties in regulating blood sugar levels, which can increase the risk of type 2 diabetes and cardiovascular disease.

A diet that focuses on low glycemic index (GI) foods, such as whole grains, fruits, vegetables, and legumes, can help stabilize blood sugar levels and improve insulin sensitivity in individuals with PCOS.

2. **Weight Management and Obesity:**
Obesity is a common comorbidity in individuals with PCOS, with up to 50-60% of affected individuals classified as overweight or obese. Excess weight can exacerbate insulin resistance, hormonal imbalances, and reproductive difficulties associated with PCOS. Therefore, weight management is an essential component of PCOS treatment. A balanced diet that emphasizes whole, nutrient-dense foods, portion control, and regular physical activity can help individuals with PCOS achieve and maintain a healthy weight.

3. **Hormonal Imbalances and Nutrient Needs:**
Hormonal imbalances, including high levels of androgens (male hormones) like testosterone, are a hallmark of PCOS. These hormone abnormalities can affect energy expenditure, appetite control,

metabolism, and energy expenditure, which can change nutrient requirements. For instance, higher protein needs may be necessary for PCOS patients to maintain hormonal balance and muscle synthesis. Furthermore, some nutrients—like magnesium, chromium, and omega-3 fatty acids—may help PCOS sufferers with their insulin sensitivity and inflammation.

4. **Gut Health and Inflammation:**
Emerging research suggests that gut health and inflammation may play a role in the pathogenesis of PCOS. Alterations in gut microbiota composition and increased intestinal permeability (leaky gut) have been observed in individuals with PCOS, which may contribute to systemic inflammation and metabolic dysfunction. A diet rich in fiber, probiotics, and anti-inflammatory foods, such as fruits, vegetables, fermented foods, and omega-3 fatty acids, may help support gut health and reduce inflammation in individuals with PCOS.

5. Psychological and Emotional Factors:
PCOS can have significant psychological and emotional effects on affected individuals, including depression, anxiety, and disordered eating behaviors. The hormonal fluctuations, menstrual irregularities, and body image concerns associated with PCOS can impact appetite, food choices, and eating patterns. Therefore, addressing the psychological and emotional aspects of PCOS alongside dietary interventions is essential for comprehensive management and improved quality of life.

Finally, it should be noted that PCOS has a significant impact on nutrition, diet, and metabolic health. As such, specialized dietary interventions are required to meet the particular requirements and difficulties faced by those who have PCOS. People with PCOS can improve their overall health outcomes and optimize their nutrition by focusing on gut health, psychological well-being, hormonal balance, blood sugar control, and weight management.

CHAPTER TWO

The PCOS Diet Approach

The PCOS diet approach is a comprehensive dietary strategy aimed at managing symptoms and improving overall health outcomes for individuals with Polycystic Ovary Syndrome (PCOS). This approach recognizes the intricate interplay between hormones, metabolism, and nutrition in PCOS and seeks to address these factors through targeted dietary interventions. By focusing on blood sugar management, hormonal balance, weight management, and nutrient optimization, the PCOS diet approach offers a holistic framework for supporting health and well-being in individuals with the condition.

1. **Emphasis on Low Glycemic Index (GI) Foods:** One of the cornerstones of the PCOS diet approach is the incorporation of low glycemic index (GI) foods. These are foods that are digested and absorbed more slowly, resulting in gradual and steady increases in blood sugar levels.

By choosing low GI foods such as whole grains, fruits, vegetables, and legumes, individuals with PCOS can help stabilize blood sugar levels, improve insulin sensitivity, and reduce the risk of insulin resistance and type 2 diabetes.

2. **Balanced Macronutrient Ratios:**
The PCOS diet approach emphasizes the importance of balanced macronutrient ratios, including adequate protein, healthy fats, and complex carbohydrates. Protein-rich foods such as lean meats, poultry, fish, tofu, and legumes provide essential amino acids for muscle synthesis and hormone production. Healthy fats from sources such as avocados, nuts, seeds, and olive oil help reduce inflammation, support hormonal balance, and promote satiety. Complex carbohydrates from whole grains, fruits, vegetables, and legumes provide sustained energy and fiber for digestion and gut health.

3. **Portion Control and Caloric Balance:**

While macronutrient quality is important, so too is portion control and caloric balance. Excess calorie consumption can contribute to weight gain, exacerbate insulin resistance, and worsen metabolic dysfunction in individuals with PCOS. Therefore, portion control and mindful eating practices are encouraged to help individuals with PCOS maintain a healthy weight and optimize metabolic health.

4. **Nutrient-Dense Foods:**

The PCOS diet approach prioritizes nutrient-dense foods that provide essential vitamins, minerals, and antioxidants to support overall health and well-being. This includes a variety of colorful fruits and vegetables, which are rich in vitamins, minerals, and phytonutrients that promote immune function, reduce inflammation, and support hormone metabolism. Additionally, lean proteins, healthy fats, and whole grains provide essential nutrients for cellular function, energy production, and hormone synthesis.

5. **Meal Timing and Frequency:**
Optimal meal timing and frequency may also play a role in managing PCOS symptoms. Some individuals with PCOS may benefit from consuming smaller, more frequent meals throughout the day to help stabilize blood sugar levels and maintain energy levels. Others may find success with intermittent fasting or time-restricted eating patterns, which have been shown to improve insulin sensitivity and metabolic health in some individuals with PCOS.

6. **Individualized Approach:**
It's important to recognize that there is no one-size-fits-all approach to the PCOS diet. Each individual may have unique dietary needs, preferences, and tolerances, and therefore, the PCOS diet approach should be tailored to meet these individual needs. Consulting with a registered dietitian or healthcare provider who specializes in PCOS can provide personalized guidance and support in developing a dietary plan that is effective and sustainable for managing PCOS symptoms.

Principles of a PCOS-friendly diet

A diet plan designed especially to meet the special requirements and difficulties faced by people with Polycystic Ovary Syndrome (PCOS) is known as a PCOS-friendly diet. A PCOS-friendly diet provides an improved way to manage symptoms and promote blood sugar control, hormonal balance, weight control, and overall well-being by emphasizing essential principles. The following are the cornerstones of a diet suitable for people with PCOS:

1. **Embrace Low Glycemic Index (GI) Foods:** Low glycemic index (GI) foods are digested and absorbed slowly, resulting in gradual and steady increases in blood sugar levels. Incorporating low GI foods such as whole grains, fruits, vegetables, and legumes into your diet can help stabilize blood sugar levels, reduce insulin resistance, and improve metabolic health in individuals with PCOS.

2. **Prioritize Protein-Rich Foods:**

Protein plays a crucial role in PCOS management, as it supports muscle synthesis, hormone production, and satiety. Including protein-rich foods such as lean meats, poultry, fish, tofu, tempeh, legumes, and Greek yogurt in your meals and snacks can help balance blood sugar levels, reduce cravings, and support weight management in individuals with PCOS.

3. **Option for Healthy Fats:**

Healthy fats are an essential component of a PCOS-friendly diet, as they provide essential fatty acids, support hormone production, and promote satiety. Choose sources of healthy fats such as avocados, nuts, seeds, olive oil, fatty fish (like salmon and mackerel), and coconut oil to incorporate into your meals and snacks.

4. Include Fiber-Rich Foods:

Fiber is important for digestive health, blood sugar regulation, and satiety, making it a valuable addition to a PCOS-friendly diet. Aim to include plenty of fiber-rich foods such as fruits, vegetables, whole grains, legumes, nuts, and seeds in your meals and snacks to support gut health and stabilize blood sugar levels.

5. Balance Carbohydrates:

While carbohydrates are an important source of energy, balancing carbohydrate intake is key for individuals with PCOS. Choose complex carbohydrates such as whole grains, fruits, vegetables, and legumes, which are rich in fiber and nutrients, over refined carbohydrates and sugary snacks, which can spike blood sugar levels and exacerbate insulin resistance.

6. Practice Portion Control:

Portion control is essential for managing calorie intake and supporting weight management in individuals with PCOS. Be mindful of portion sizes and listen to your body's hunger and fullness cues to avoid overeating. Using smaller plates, measuring serving sizes, and paying attention to portion sizes when dining out can help you maintain control over your food intake.

7. **Stay Hydrated:**
Proper hydration is important for overall health and well-being, including hormone balance and metabolic function. Aim to drink plenty of water throughout the day and limit sugary beverages and caffeinated drinks, which can disrupt blood sugar levels and exacerbate hormonal imbalances in individuals with PCOS.

8. **Limit Processed Foods and Added Sugars:**
Processed foods and added sugars should be limited in a PCOS-friendly diet, as they can contribute to inflammation, insulin resistance, and weight gain. Instead, focus on whole, minimally processed foods that are nutrient-dense and support optimal health and well-being.

In summary, the foundation of a PCOS-friendly diet is a set of ideas that promote hormonal balance, weight control, blood sugar regulation, and general health. People with PCOS can improve their nutrition and quality of life by adopting low-GI foods, giving priority to foods high in protein and fiber, controlling portion sizes, balancing carbs, drinking plenty of water, and avoiding processed and added sugars. A registered dietitian or other PCOS-specialized healthcare professional can offer individualized advice and support in putting these dietary guidelines into practice and achieving long-term success in managing PCOS symptoms.

Macronutrient balance: carbs, proteins, and fats

Achieving a balanced macronutrient intake is crucial for individuals with Polycystic Ovary Syndrome (PCOS) to manage symptoms, support hormonal balance, and promote overall health and well-being. A well-rounded PCOS diet focuses on optimizing the intake of carbohydrates, proteins, and fats to address the unique metabolic and hormonal challenges associated with the condition.

1. Carbohydrates:

Carbohydrates are the body's primary source of energy and play a significant role in blood sugar management, which is particularly important for individuals with PCOS who may experience insulin resistance. When choosing carbohydrates in the PCOS diet, the focus is on selecting complex carbohydrates with a low glycemic index (GI) that are digested and absorbed more slowly, leading to gradual increases in blood sugar levels and improved insulin sensitivity.

Examples of PCOS-friendly complex carbohydrates include:
Whole grains include barley, brown rice, quinoa, oats, and whole wheat.
Fruits such as berries, apples, pears, and citrus fruits
Vegetables such as leafy greens, broccoli, cauliflower, carrots, and bell peppers.
Legumes like kidney beans, black beans, chickpeas, and lentils.
In the PCOS diet, limiting the consumption of refined carbohydrates and sugary snacks is also crucial to avoid blood sugar spikes and an aggravation of insulin resistance.

2. Proteins:

Proteins are essential for supporting muscle synthesis, hormone production, and satiety, making them a key component of the PCOS diet. Including adequate protein in meals and snacks helps stabilize blood sugar levels, reduce cravings, and support weight management in individuals with PCOS.

Sources of PCOS-friendly proteins include:
Lean meats such as poultry (chicken, turkey) and lean cuts of beef or pork
Fish such as salmon, trout, tuna, and tilapia
Plant-based proteins such as tofu, tempeh, edamame, and legumes (lentils, chickpeas, black beans)
Dairy or dairy alternatives such as Greek yogurt, cottage cheese, and unsweetened almond or soy milk
Balancing protein intake throughout the day and including protein-rich foods in each meal and snack can help individuals with PCOS feel satisfied, maintain muscle mass, and support hormonal balance.

3. **Fats:**
Healthy fats are essential for hormone production, cell membrane function, and nutrient absorption, making them an important component of the PCOS diet. Including sources of healthy fats in moderation helps reduce inflammation, support hormone

balance, and promote satiety in individuals with
PCOS.

**Sources of good fats that are suitable for PCOS
include:**
Avocados
Nuts and seeds, including flaxseeds, chia seeds,
walnuts, and almonds
Olive oil.
fatty fish, including trout, sardines, salmon, and
mackerel. Coconut lubricant
To lower inflammation and promote cardiovascular
health, limiting the consumption of saturated and
trans fats—found in processed foods, fried foods,
and fatty meats—is another crucial component of
the PCOS diet.

In summary, maintaining a balanced intake of
macronutrients is critical for PCOS sufferers to
control their symptoms, maintain hormonal balance,
and advance their general health and wellbeing.
People with PCOS can improve their quality of life
and optimize their nutrition by emphasizing low-GI
complex carbohydrates, enough protein, and
moderate amounts of healthy fats. Using a balanced
macronutrient approach to the PCOS diet can be

made easier by working with a registered dietitian or other healthcare professional who specializes in PCOS.

Importance of fiber and micronutrients

When it comes to managing Polycystic Ovary Syndrome (PCOS), macronutrients such as proteins, fats, and carbohydrates are frequently the focus of attention. But fiber and micronutrients are just as important; they are critical for maintaining hormone balance, metabolic health, and general well-being in PCOS patients. This is a thorough examination of the role that fiber and micronutrients play in the PCOS diet:

1. **Fiber**:

Blood Sugar Management: Fiber-rich foods have a remarkable ability to modulate blood sugar levels by slowing down the absorption of glucose into the bloodstream. This is particularly beneficial for individuals with PCOS who may struggle with insulin resistance and elevated blood sugar levels. By promoting more stable blood sugar levels, fiber helps alleviate symptoms associated with PCOS and reduces the risk of developing type 2 diabetes.

Weight Management: Fiber contributes to feelings of fullness and satiety, which can aid in weight management by reducing overall calorie intake and curbing cravings. For individuals with PCOS, maintaining a healthy weight is crucial for managing symptoms and improving metabolic health. By promoting feelings of fullness, fiber-rich foods can support weight loss efforts and contribute to long-term weight management.

Digestive Health: Fiber plays a key role in digestive health by promoting regular bowel movements, preventing constipation, and supporting a healthy gut microbiome. A healthy gut microbiome is essential for overall health and has been linked to improved metabolic function, reduced inflammation, and enhanced immune function. By incorporating fiber-rich foods into the diet, individuals with PCOS can support digestive health and optimize their overall well-being.

2. **Micronutrients:**

Hormone Balance: Micronutrients such as vitamins and minerals are essential for hormone production, metabolism, and regulation. In individuals with PCOS, micronutrient deficiencies can disrupt hormone balance and exacerbate symptoms of the condition. For example, deficiencies in vitamins D and B12 have been associated with insulin resistance and hormonal imbalances in individuals with PCOS. By ensuring adequate intake of micronutrients through a balanced diet, individuals with PCOS can support hormone balance and metabolic function.

Nutrient Absorption: Micronutrients play a crucial role in nutrient absorption and utilization within the body. Certain micronutrients, such as vitamin C and iron, enhance the absorption of other nutrients, such as iron and calcium. Ensuring adequate intake of micronutrients is essential for optimal nutrient absorption and utilization, which is particularly important for individuals with PCOS who may have increased nutrient needs or absorption challenges.

Reduced Inflammation: Many micronutrients possess anti-inflammatory properties and play a role in reducing oxidative stress and inflammation within the body. Chronic inflammation is a common feature of PCOS and has been implicated in the development of insulin resistance, hormonal imbalances, and other metabolic disturbances. By incorporating micronutrient-rich foods into the diet, individuals with PCOS can help reduce inflammation and support overall health.

In summary, fiber and micronutrients are critical elements of a PCOS diet that promote hormone balance, metabolic health, and general wellbeing. People with PCOS can improve their quality of life and optimize their nutrition by giving priority to foods high in fiber and micronutrients, such as fruits, vegetables, whole grains, nuts, and seeds, as well as lean proteins. A registered dietitian or other PCOS-specialized healthcare professional can offer individualized advice and support on how to include fiber and micronutrients in the diet to effectively manage symptoms and enhance long-term health outcomes.

CHAPTER THREE

Meal Planning and Preparation

Organizing and preparing meals well is essential to controlling Polycystic Ovary Syndrome (PCOS) with food. People with PCOS can manage their symptoms, enhance overall health, and optimize their nutrition by carefully choosing nutrient-dense foods, balancing macronutrients, and adding fiber and micronutrients. This is an all-inclusive meal planning and preparation guide for the PCOS diet:

1. **Set Clear Goals**: It's important to establish clear goals based on personal needs, preferences, and health objectives before beginning the meal planning process. Setting clear, attainable goals will direct the process of meal planning and guarantee success, regardless of the objective—stabilizing

blood sugar, assisting with weight management, or enhancing hormone balance, for example.

2. Choose Nutrient-Dense Foods:
Focus on selecting nutrient-dense foods that provide a wide range of vitamins, minerals, and antioxidants to support overall health and well-being. Incorporate a variety of colorful fruits and vegetables, lean proteins, whole grains, healthy fats, and legumes into meals and snacks to ensure a balanced and nutritious diet.

3. Balance Macronutrients:
Pay attention to macronutrient balance by including a combination of carbohydrates, proteins, and fats in each meal and snack. Aim for a balanced ratio of macronutrients to support blood sugar management, satiety, and hormone balance. For example, pair complex carbohydrates with lean proteins and healthy fats to create satisfying and balanced meals.

4. Emphasize Fiber-Rich Foods:

Incorporate fiber-rich foods such as fruits, vegetables, whole grains, nuts, seeds, and legumes into meals and snacks to support digestive health, stabilize blood sugar levels, and promote satiety.

Aim to include a variety of fiber-rich foods throughout the day to meet daily fiber recommendations and support overall well-being.

5. **Plan Ahead:** Give yourself enough time to organize your weekly menu, taking into account things like dietary restrictions, social obligations, and work schedules. Make a weekly meal plan with a range of nutrient-dense foods and recipes, ensuring that each meal includes foods high in fiber, lean proteins, and healthy fats.

6. **Batch Cooking and Meal Prep**: To expedite the cooking process and save time during hectic weekdays, dedicate time to meal preparation at the start of the week. Think about preparing basic ingredients in bulk, like grains, proteins, and veggies, as they can serve as the foundation for preparing quick and simple meals all week long.

Meal planning and portion control can be facilitated by preparing meals ahead of time and dividing them into individual serving containers.

7. **Stock Up on Healthy Staples:**

Keep a well-stocked pantry, refrigerator, and freezer with healthy staples such as whole grains, lean proteins, fruits, vegetables, nuts, seeds, and healthy fats. Having these ingredients on hand makes it easier to whip up nutritious meals and snacks at a moment's notice, reducing the temptation to rely on processed or convenience foods.

8. **Be Flexible and Adaptable**: When it comes to meal planning and preparation, be flexible and adaptable. Modify recipes and menus as necessary to account for shifting dietary needs, schedules, and preferences. To keep meals interesting and fun, try different flavors, ingredients, and cooking methods. You can also get ideas for new recipes by browsing cookbooks, websites, and social media.

To sum up, meal preparation and planning are crucial aspects of the PCOS diet that promote healthy eating, symptom control, and general wellbeing. People with PCOS can develop a sustainable and enjoyable eating strategy that supports health and happiness by setting clear goals, selecting nutrient-dense foods, balancing macronutrients, highlighting fiber-rich foods, planning ahead, batch cooking, stockpiling healthy staples, and remaining flexible and adaptable. Developing successful meal plans and success strategies can be aided by consulting with a registered dietitian or other healthcare professional who specializes in PCOS.

Tips for meal planning with PCOS in mind

Meal planning with PCOS in mind requires careful consideration of nutrient balance, portion control, and managing symptoms associated with the condition. Here are comprehensive tips for effective meal planning with PCOS:

Set Clear Goals: Determine specific health goals related to PCOS management, such as stabilizing blood sugar levels, supporting weight management, or improving hormone balance.

Prioritize Nutrient-Dense Foods: Choose whole, nutrient-dense foods that provide essential vitamins, minerals, and antioxidants to support overall health and well-being.

Balance Macronutrients: Aim for a balanced ratio of carbohydrates, proteins, and fats in each meal to support blood sugar management, satiety, and hormone balance.

Focus on Fiber: Incorporate fiber-rich foods such as fruits, vegetables, whole grains, nuts, seeds, and legumes to support digestive health, stabilize blood sugar levels, and promote satiety.

Plan Ahead: Take time to plan meals and snacks for the week ahead, considering factors such as work schedules, social commitments, and dietary preferences.

Batch Cooking: Spend time on meal preparation at the beginning of the week by batch cooking staple ingredients that can be used as building blocks for creating quick and easy meals.

Portion Control: Practice portion control to prevent overeating and support weight management. Use smaller plates, measuring cups, and portioning tools to help control portion sizes.

Include Lean Proteins: Choose lean sources of protein such as poultry, fish, tofu, tempeh, legumes, and Greek yogurt to support muscle synthesis, hormone balance, and satiety.

Incorporate Healthy Fats: Include sources of healthy fats such as avocados, nuts, seeds, olive oil, and fatty fish to support hormone production, cell membrane function, and satiety.

Limit Processed Foods: Minimize the consumption of processed foods, sugary snacks, and refined carbohydrates, which can exacerbate insulin resistance and hormonal imbalances.

Keep Yourself Hydrated: To maintain general health and stay hydrated, sip lots of water throughout the day. Restrict your intake of sugary and caffeinated drinks as they can upset your hormone balance and blood sugar levels.

Experiment with Recipes: Try new recipes and cooking techniques to keep meals exciting and enjoyable. Look for PCOS-friendly recipes that prioritize whole, nutrient-dense ingredients.

Include Prebiotic Foods: Incorporate prebiotic foods such as onions, garlic, leeks, asparagus, and bananas to support gut health and promote a healthy microbiome.

Eat mindfully by paying attention to your body's signals of hunger and fullness, and by eating slowly to aid in digestion and avoid overindulging. Steer clear of distractions like screens and fast food.

Seek Support: Connect with a registered dietitian or healthcare provider who specializes in PCOS to receive personalized guidance and support in developing effective meal plans and strategies for success.

Track Your Progress: Analyze your eating patterns, symptoms, and advancement toward your objectives to spot trends and make necessary corrections. Reevaluate objectives and tactics on a regular basis to guarantee that diet-based PCOS management remains successful.

These pointers can help you develop a sustainable and successful eating strategy that supports PCOS management and enhances general health and wellbeing. Simply incorporate them into your meal planning routine.

Strategies for grocery shopping and ingredient selection

It can be intimidating to navigate the grocery store aisles, particularly if you're on a PCOS diet or another restrictive diet. In order to facilitate PCOS management and enhance the efficiency of grocery shopping, take into account the following extensive strategies when choosing ingredients:

1. **Create a List**: Based on your meal plan and dietary preferences, create a list of PCOS-friendly foods and ingredients before you go to the grocery store. This will assist you in maintaining focus and preventing impulsive purchases of less wholesome goods.

2. **Plan Meals in Advance**: Plan your meals for the week ahead of time, including breakfast, lunch, dinner, and snacks. This will give you a clear idea of what ingredients you need to purchase and prevent last-minute decisions that may not align with your PCOS diet goals.

3. **Choose Whole, Nutrient-Dense Foods**: Focus on selecting whole, nutrient-dense foods that provide essential vitamins, minerals, and antioxidants to support overall health and well-being. Opt for fresh fruits and vegetables, whole grains, lean proteins, healthy fats, and legumes whenever possible.

4. **Prioritize Fresh Produce**: Load up on a variety of colorful fruits and vegetables, which are rich in fiber, vitamins, and minerals. Aim to include a rainbow of colors in your cart to ensure a diverse intake of nutrients that support PCOS management.

5. **Read Labels Carefully**: Pay attention to food labels and ingredient lists to identify hidden sugars,

additives, and preservatives that may negatively impact PCOS symptoms. Choose minimally processed foods with simple, recognizable ingredients and avoid products with added sugars, artificial sweeteners, and trans fats.

6. **Option for Lean Proteins**: Choose lean sources of protein such as skinless poultry, fish, tofu, tempeh, legumes, and Greek yogurt. Look for grass-fed and organic options when possible to minimize exposure to hormones and antibiotics.

7. **Incorporate Healthy Fats**: Include sources of healthy fats such as avocados, nuts, seeds, olive oil, and fatty fish in your shopping cart. These fats are essential for hormone production, cell membrane function, and satiety, making them important components of the PCOS diet.

8. **Stock Up on Whole Grains**: Choose whole grains such as brown rice, quinoa, oats, barley, and

whole wheat bread and pasta to provide fiber, vitamins, and minerals. These complex carbohydrates help stabilize blood sugar levels and support digestive health.

9. **Include Plant-Based Proteins**: Incorporate plant-based protein sources such as beans, lentils, chickpeas, and tofu into your shopping list to add variety and diversity to your meals. Plant-based proteins are rich in fiber and phytonutrients and can help support PCOS management.

10. **Avoid Highly Processed Foods**: Limit the purchase of highly processed foods, sugary snacks, and refined carbohydrates, which can contribute to insulin resistance and hormonal imbalances. Stick to the perimeter of the grocery store where fresh, whole foods are typically located.

11. **Consider Frozen and Canned Options**: Don't overlook frozen and canned fruits and vegetables,

which can be convenient and cost-effective alternatives to fresh produce. Just be sure to choose options without added sugars, sauces, or preservatives.

12. **Stock Up on Herbs and Spices**: Enhance the flavor of your meals without adding extra calories or sodium by stocking up on herbs, spices, and seasoning blends. Experiment with different flavors and cuisines to keep your meals interesting and enjoyable.

13. **Be Mindful of Portions:** Pay attention to portion sizes when selecting packaged foods, especially snacks and convenience items. Opt for single-serving portions or portion out larger packages into smaller containers to prevent overeating.

14. **Check for Sales and Discounts**: Keep an eye out for sales, discounts, and coupons on

PCOS-friendly foods and ingredients to save money while supporting your dietary goals. Consider buying in bulk or stocking up on non-perishable items when they're on sale.

15. **Stay Hydrated:** Don't forget to include beverages like water, herbal tea, and unsweetened almond milk on your shopping list to stay hydrated throughout the week. Limit sugary drinks, sodas, and fruit juices, which can contribute to blood sugar spikes and insulin resistance.

By incorporating these strategies into your grocery shopping routine, you can make informed choices that support PCOS management and promote overall health and well-being. Remember to stay flexible and adapt your shopping list based on your individual preferences, dietary needs, and lifestyle considerations.

Batch cooking and meal prep techniques

Batch cooking and meal prep are invaluable strategies for individuals managing Polycystic Ovary Syndrome (PCOS) through diet. These techniques not only save time and energy but also ensure that nutritious meals are readily available, making it easier to adhere to the PCOS-friendly eating plan. Here's a comprehensive guide to batch cooking and meal prep for the PCOS diet:

1. **Plan Your Meals**: To begin, arrange your meals for the upcoming week. When making your meal plan, take your nutritional requirements, dietary

preferences, and schedule into account. Try to find a range of recipes that are good for PCOS and include whole grains, lean proteins, healthy fats, and an abundance of fruits and vegetables.

2. **Choose Recipes Wisely**:
Select recipes that lend themselves well to batch cooking and meal prep. Dishes such as soups, stews, casseroles, stir-fries, and grain bowls are excellent options as they can be easily prepared in large quantities and reheated throughout the week.

3. **Make a Grocery List:**
Once you've chosen your recipes, make a comprehensive grocery list of all the ingredients you'll need. This will help streamline your shopping trip and ensure that you have everything on hand when it's time to start cooking.

4. **Schedule a Cooking Day:**

Set aside a designated day each week for batch cooking and meal prep. This could be a weekend day or a day when you have some extra time available. Block off a few hours in your schedule to focus solely on cooking and preparing meals for the week ahead.

5. **Prepare Your Ingredients**: Give your ingredients some thought before you begin cooking. Prepare grains and legumes into portion sizes, wash and chop fruits and vegetables, and marinate proteins as needed. Making sure everything is prepared and ready to go will greatly streamline the cooking process.

6. **Cook in Batches:**
Once your ingredients are prepped, start cooking your meals in batches. Use large pots, pans, and baking dishes to prepare multiple servings at once. This will save time and energy compared to cooking each meal individually.

7. **Utilize Time-Saving Appliances:**
Make use of time-saving appliances such as slow cookers, instant pots, and rice cookers to streamline the cooking process. These appliances allow you to set it and forget it, freeing up time to focus on other tasks while your meals cook.

8. **Portion Out Meals:**
Once your meals are cooked, portion them out into individual containers for easy grab-and-go access throughout the week. Use meal prep containers with compartments to keep different components of the meal separate and prevent them from getting soggy.

9. **Label and Store:** Make sure to write the dish's name and preparation date on the labels of your containers. By doing this, you can make sure that you're eating meals while they're still fresh and keep track of what's in your refrigerator. Meals should be kept in the freezer or refrigerator depending on when you intend to eat them.

10. **Mix and Match Components**:
To keep meals interesting, mix and match different components throughout the week. For example, pair a protein from one meal with a grain and vegetable from another meal to create a new dish. This allows for variety while still utilizing the meals you've prepared.

11. **Incorporate Quick and Easy Snacks:**
In addition to main meals, batch cook and prepare quick and easy snacks such as cut-up fruits and vegetables, hard-boiled eggs, yogurt parfaits, and trail mix. Having healthy snacks on hand will help curb cravings and prevent reaching for less nutritious options.

12. **Stay Organized:**
Keep your refrigerator and pantry organized to make it easy to find what you need. Store batch-cooked meals and prepped ingredients in clear, labeled containers at eye level for quick access.

13. **Reheat Safely:**
When reheating meals, be sure to do so safely to prevent foodborne illness. Use a microwave, stovetop, or oven to reheat meals until they reach an internal temperature of 165°F (74°C) before consuming.

14. **Experiment and Adapt:**
Don't be afraid to experiment with different recipes, ingredients, and cooking techniques to keep meals exciting and enjoyable. Adapt your meal prep routine based on your preferences, dietary needs, and lifestyle considerations.

15. **Stay Consistent:**
Consistency is key when it comes to batch cooking and meal prep. Make it a regular part of your routine to set yourself up for success in managing PCOS through diet.

You can simplify nutrition, save time, and make it simpler to follow the PCOS-friendly eating plan by implementing these batch cooking and meal prep techniques into your daily routine. All it takes is a little planning and preparation to have wholesome and tasty meals ready for the entire week.

CHAPTER FOUR

Breakfast Recipes

Breakfast is an important meal, especially for individuals managing Polycystic Ovary Syndrome (PCOS). Starting the day with a balanced and nutritious meal can help stabilize blood sugar levels, support hormone balance, and provide sustained energy throughout the morning. Here are several PCOS diet-friendly breakfast recipes to kickstart your day on a healthy note:

1. Greek Yogurt Parfait:

1/2 cup plain Greek yogurt

1/4 cup mixed berries (such as strawberries, blueberries, and raspberries)

1 tablespoon chia seeds

1 tablespoon sliced almonds

Drizzle of honey or maple syrup (optional)

Layer Greek yogurt, mixed berries, chia seeds, and sliced almonds in a glass or bowl. Drizzle with honey or maple syrup if desired. Enjoy this protein-rich parfait packed with fiber, vitamins, and antioxidants.

2. **Veggie Omelette:**

Two big eggs

1/4 cup finely chopped veggies, including tomatoes, onions, bell peppers, and spinach

One tablespoon of shredded cheese, if desired

To taste, add salt and pepper.

In a bowl, whisk together eggs and add pepper and salt to taste. Pour the beaten eggs into a nonstick skillet that has been heated to medium heat. On one side of the omelet, place the cheese and chopped vegetables after cooking for a few minutes or until the edges begin to set. Once the cheese has melted, fold the other side over the filling and continue cooking for a minute. Serve warm, accompanied by avocado slices or whole grain toast on the side.

3. Overnight Oats:
1/2 cup rolled oats
1/2 cup unsweetened almond milk
1/4 cup Greek yogurt
1 tablespoon chia seeds
1/2 teaspoon vanilla extract
1 tablespoon nut butter (such as almond or peanut butter)
Sliced banana and berries for topping

In a jar or container, combine rolled oats, almond milk, Greek yogurt, chia seeds, vanilla extract, and nut butter. Stir well to combine, then cover and refrigerate overnight. In the morning, top with sliced banana and berries for added sweetness and fiber.

4. Avocado Toast with Poached Egg:
 One piece of whole grain bread
1/2 mashed, ripe avocado
One stolen egg
To taste, add salt, pepper, and red pepper flakes.

Feta cheese, microgreens, and tomato slices are optional toppings.

When the whole grain bread is golden brown, toast it. After evenly spreading the mashed avocado on the toast, season it with red pepper flakes, salt, and pepper. Add a poached egg and any other desired toppings on top. Savor this nutrient-dense breakfast that is high in fiber, protein, and healthy fats.

5. Smoothie Bowl:

One banana, frozen

Half a cup of mixed berries, including blueberries, raspberries, and strawberries

half a cup kale or spinach

Half a cup of unflavored almond milk

One tablespoon of chia seeds

sliced fruits, granola, almonds, and seeds as toppings

Blend frozen banana, mixed berries, kale or spinach, almond milk, and chia seeds in a blender. Blend until creamy and smooth. Transfer the smoothie into a bowl and garnish with granola, almonds, seeds, and sliced fruits to add more nutrients and texture. Savor this filling and revitalizing breakfast choice.

6. Quinoa Breakfast Bowl:

1/2 cup cooked quinoa
1/4 cup Greek yogurt
1 tablespoon almond butter
1/2 banana, sliced
Handful of berries
Sprinkle of cinnamon

In a bowl, layer cooked quinoa, Greek yogurt, almond butter, sliced banana, and berries. Sprinkle with cinnamon for added flavor and enjoy this protein-packed breakfast bowl that's both nourishing and satisfying.

7. Chia Seed Pudding:

Two tsp of chia seeds
Half a cup of unflavored almond milk
Half a teaspoon of extract from vanilla
Sweeteners to taste: stevia, honey, and maple syrup
Add-ons: coconut flakes, almonds, seeds, and sliced fruits

Mix the almond milk, vanilla extract, and chia seeds in a jar or other container. Once everything is well combined, cover and chill for a minimum of two hours or overnight, or until the mixture takes on the consistency of pudding. If desired, add honey, maple syrup, or stevia to taste. For extra texture and taste, sprinkle sliced fruits, nuts, seeds, and coconut flakes on top. Savor this high-fiber pudding for a filling and healthy start to the day.

Each of the PCOS diet-friendly breakfast recipes outlined offers a range of health benefits, tailored to support individuals managing Polycystic Ovary Syndrome (PCOS). Here's an explanation of the health benefits associated with each recipe:

1. **Greek Yogurt Parfait:**

Protein-Rich: Greek yogurt is a high-protein food, which helps promote satiety, stabilize blood sugar levels, and support muscle repair and growth.

Rich in Fiber: Berries and chia seeds are rich in fiber, aiding in digestion, promoting feelings of fullness, and supporting gut health.
Antioxidants: Berries are packed with antioxidants that help combat inflammation and oxidative stress, which are common in individuals with PCOS.

2. **Veggie Omelette**:

Protein and Fiber: Eggs are a complete source of protein, while vegetables like spinach and bell peppers provide fiber and essential nutrients. This combination helps stabilize blood sugar levels and supports feelings of fullness.

Nutrient-Dense: Vegetables in the omelet provide a variety of vitamins, minerals, and antioxidants, supporting overall health and well-being.

3. **Overnight Oats:**

High Fiber: Oats and chia seeds are high in fiber, promoting digestive health, regulating blood sugar levels, and supporting weight management.
Heart-Healthy Fats: Chia seeds and nut butter provide healthy fats, which are essential for

hormone production, cell membrane function, and satiety.

Customizable: Overnight oats can be customized with various toppings, allowing for versatility and personalization to suit individual tastes and preferences.

4. **Avocado Toast with Poached Egg:**

Healthy Fats: Avocado is rich in monounsaturated fats, which help reduce inflammation, support hormone balance, and promote heart health.
Protein: Eggs provide high-quality protein, which supports muscle synthesis, satiety, and hormone production.

Complex Carbohydrates: Whole grain bread provides complex carbohydrates for sustained energy release and fiber for digestive health.

5. **Smoothie Bowl:**

Nutrient-Rich: Smoothie bowls are packed with fruits, vegetables, and other nutritious ingredients, providing a wide range of vitamins, minerals, and antioxidants.

Hydration: Smoothie bowls made with almond milk and fruits contribute to hydration, supporting overall health and well-being.

Digestive Health: Spinach or kale in the smoothie bowl provides fiber, aiding in digestion and promoting gut health.

6. Quinoa Breakfast Bowl:

Complete Protein: Quinoa is a complete protein, containing all essential amino acids, which supports muscle repair and growth, hormone balance, and satiety.

Healthy Fats: Almond butter provides healthy fats, which support hormone production, cell membrane function, and satiety.

Complex Carbohydrates: Quinoa provides complex carbohydrates for sustained energy release and fiber for digestive health.

7. Chia Seed Pudding:

Omega-3 Fatty Acids: Chia seeds are rich in omega-3 fatty acids, which have anti-inflammatory properties and support heart health, brain function, and hormone balance.

High Fiber: Chia seeds are high in fiber, promoting digestive health, regulating blood sugar levels, and supporting weight management.
Versatile: Chia seed pudding can be customized with various toppings, allowing for versatility and personalization to suit individual tastes and preferences.

In summary, each of these PCOS diet-friendly breakfast recipes offers a combination of protein, fiber, healthy fats, vitamins, minerals, and antioxidants to support overall health and well-being. By incorporating these nutrient-rich options into your morning routine, you can start your day off on the right foot and better manage symptoms associated with PCOS.

Nutrient-rich breakfast options to kickstart your day

Starting your day with a nutrient-rich breakfast is essential for individuals managing Polycystic Ovary Syndrome (PCOS). A well-balanced breakfast provides the energy and nutrients needed to support hormone balance, stabilize blood sugar levels, and promote overall well-being. Here are several comprehensive options for nutrient-rich breakfasts tailored to the PCOS diet:

1. Greek Yogurt Bowl with Mixed Berries and Nuts:

Ingredients:
1/2 cup plain Greek yogurt
1/4 cup mixed berries (such as strawberries, blueberries, and raspberries).
One tablespoon of finely chopped nuts, like pecans, walnuts, or almonds.
Drizzle of honey or sprinkle of cinnamon (optional).

Health Benefits:

High in Protein: Greek yogurt provides a significant amount of protein, which supports muscle repair and growth, promotes satiety, and helps stabilize blood sugar levels.
Rich in Antioxidants: Berries are loaded with antioxidants, including vitamins C and E, which

help combat inflammation, oxidative stress, and cellular damage.

Healthy Fats: Nuts are a good source of healthy fats, including omega-3 fatty acids, which support heart health, hormone production, and brain function.

Customizable: This breakfast option is highly customizable, allowing for variations in fruit selection, nut choice, and optional toppings like honey or cinnamon.

2. Spinach and Feta Breakfast Wrap:

Ingredients:
1 whole grain wrap or tortilla
2 large eggs, scrambled
Handful of fresh spinach leaves
1 tablespoon crumbled feta cheese
Sliced tomato and avocado (optional).

Health Benefits:

Protein-Packed: Eggs provide high-quality protein, essential for muscle synthesis, satiety, and hormone balance.

Iron and Folate: Spinach is rich in iron and folate, supporting red blood cell production, energy metabolism, and reproductive health.

Calcium: Feta cheese provides calcium, which is important for bone health and muscle function.

Whole Grains: Whole grain wrap or tortilla offers complex carbohydrates and fiber for sustained energy release and digestive health.

3. Quinoa Breakfast Bowl with Fruit and Almonds:

Ingredients:
1/2 cup cooked quinoa
1/4 cup sliced mixed fruits (such as banana, berries, and mango)
1 tablespoon sliced almonds
Drizzle of honey or sprinkle of cinnamon (optional).

Health Benefits:

Complete Protein: Quinoa is a complete protein, containing all essential amino acids, which supports muscle repair and growth, hormone balance, and satiety.

Fiber-Rich: Quinoa and fruits provide fiber, aiding in digestion, regulating blood sugar levels, and promoting satiety.

Healthy Fats: Almonds are a good source of healthy fats, including monounsaturated fats and omega-3 fatty acids, which support heart health, brain function, and hormone production.

Antioxidants: Fruits are rich in antioxidants, vitamins, and minerals, which help combat inflammation, oxidative stress, and cellular damage.

4. Smoked Salmon and Avocado Toast:

Ingredients:

1 slice whole grain bread, toasted

1/4 ripe avocado, mashed

2 ounces smoked salmon

Sliced cucumber and red onion (optional).

Health Benefits:

Omega-3 Fatty Acids: Smoked salmon is rich in omega-3 fatty acids, which have anti-inflammatory

properties and support heart health, brain function, and hormone balance.
Healthy Fats: Avocado provides monounsaturated fats, which support hormone production, cell membrane function, and satiety.
Lean Protein: Smoked salmon is a lean source of protein, essential for muscle repair and growth, satiety, and hormone balance.
Complex Carbohydrates: Whole grain bread offers complex carbohydrates and fiber for sustained energy release and digestive health.

5. Berry and Green Smoothie:

Ingredients:
Half a cup of mixed berries, including blueberries, raspberries, and strawberries
handful of kale or spinach
half a banana
One tablespoon of chia seeds
a cup of almond milk without sugar.

Health Benefits:

Antioxidants: Berries and leafy greens are rich in antioxidants, vitamins, and minerals, which help combat inflammation, oxidative stress, and cellular damage.

Fiber-Rich: Berries, banana, and chia seeds provide fiber, aiding in digestion, regulating blood sugar levels, and promoting satiety.

Hydration: Smoothies made with almond milk and fruits contribute to hydration, supporting overall health and well-being.

Customizable: This breakfast option is highly customizable, allowing for variations in fruit selection, leafy greens, and optional additions like protein powder or nut butter.

By including these nutrient-dense breakfast options in your daily routine, you can support overall health and well-being while managing PCOS by getting essential vitamins, minerals, antioxidants, protein, healthy fats, and fiber. Try a variety of ingredients, flavors, and textures to determine which combinations work best for your dietary requirements and taste preferences.

Quick and easy breakfast recipes for busy mornings

For individuals managing Polycystic Ovary Syndrome (PCOS), busy mornings can make it challenging to prioritize a nutritious breakfast. However, starting the day with a balanced meal is essential for stabilizing blood sugar levels, supporting hormone balance, and promoting overall well-being. Here are several quick and easy breakfast recipes tailored to the PCOS diet:

1. Berry Overnight Oats:

Ingredients:
1/2 cup rolled oats
1/2 cup unsweetened almond milk
1/4 cup mixed berries (such as strawberries, blueberries, and raspberries)
1 tablespoon chia seeds
Drizzle of honey or maple syrup (optional).

Instructions:

Rollin oats, almond milk, mixed berries, and chia seeds should all be combined in a jar or container. After giving everything a good stir, cover and chill for the night.
Stir the oats briefly in the morning and serve cold, or reheat in the microwave if preferred.
If desired, drizzle with maple syrup or honey for extra sweetness.

2. Spinach and Feta Egg Muffins:

Ingredients:
6 large eggs
1 cup chopped spinach
1/4 cup crumbled feta cheese
Salt and pepper to taste.

Instructions:
Set a muffin tin to lightly grease and preheat the oven to 350°F (175°C).
Beat eggs, feta cheese, chopped spinach, salt, and pepper in a bowl.
Using an even pouring motion, fill each muffin cup about 3/4 of the way to the top.

Bake for 15 to 20 minutes, or until the egg muffins are set and have a light golden color, in a preheated oven.

Before taking the muffins out of the tin, let them cool slightly. For convenient grab-and-go breakfasts throughout the week, serve warm or keep chilled.

3. Greek Yogurt Smoothie:

Ingredients:
Half a cup of Greek yogurt, plain
Half a cup of mixed berries, including blueberries, raspberries, and strawberries
half a banana
One tablespoon of peanut butter or almond butter
Almond milk (1/2 cup, unsweetened).

Instructions:
Greek yogurt, mixed berries, banana, almond butter, and almond milk should all be combined in a blender.
To get the right consistency, add extra almond milk if necessary and blend until smooth and creamy. Immediately pour the smoothie into a glass and enjoy it, or transfer it to a travel-friendly container for an easy on-the-go breakfast.

4. Avocado Toast with Hard-Boiled Egg:

Ingredients:
One quarter of a ripe avocado, one hard-boiled egg, one slice of whole grain bread, and salt, pepper, and red pepper flakes to taste.

Instructions:
Over the toasted whole grain bread, equally distribute the mashed avocado.
Spoon a hard-boiled egg slice over the avocado.
To taste, add more pepper, salt, and red pepper flakes for seasoning.
Serve right away for a simple and filling breakfast choice.

5. Peanut Butter Banana Wrap:

Ingredients:
1 whole grain wrap or tortilla
2 tablespoons peanut butter
1/2 banana, sliced.

Instructions:

Evenly spread peanut butter over the tortilla or whole grain wrapper.

Place the sliced banana over the peanut butter layer.

Tightly roll the wrap, cut in half, and serve right away for a simple and portable breakfast choice.

6. Chia Seed Pudding Parfait:

Ingredients:

Two tsp of chia seeds

Half a cup of unflavored almond milk

Half a cup of mixed berries, including blueberries, raspberries, and strawberries

Two tablespoons of crushed nuts or granola.

Instructions:

Mix the almond milk and chia seeds in a jar or other container. Mix thoroughly to blend.

Cover and chill until the mixture thickens and takes on the consistency of pudding, which should take at least two hours or overnight.

Make a parfait in the morning by layering chia seed pudding, mixed berries, and either crushed nuts or granola in a glass or bowl.

Serve right away for a simple and wholesome breakfast choice.

7. Veggie Breakfast Wrap:

Ingredients:
1 whole grain wrap or tortilla
2 scrambled eggs
Handful of baby spinach leaves
Sliced tomato and avocado.

Instructions:
Prepare scrambled eggs in a skillet until cooked through.
Warm the whole grain wrap or tortilla in the skillet or microwave.
Layer scrambled eggs, baby spinach leaves, sliced tomato, and avocado on the wrap.
Roll up the wrap tightly, slice in half if desired, and serve immediately for a quick and satisfying breakfast option.

Low glycemic index breakfast ideas

Those who manage Polycystic Ovary Syndrome (PCOS) must maintain stable blood sugar levels; selecting breakfast foods with a low GI can assist in achieving this objective. Low GI foods improve insulin sensitivity and cause blood sugar levels to rise gradually because they are absorbed and digested more slowly. The following are a few thorough low-GI breakfast suggestions suited to the PCOS diet:

1. Vegetable Omelet with Whole Grain Toast:

Ingredients:
2 large eggs
Handful of chopped vegetables (such as spinach, bell peppers, onions, and mushrooms)
1 slice whole grain toast.

Instructions:
In a bowl, whisk together eggs and add pepper and salt to taste.
Pour the beaten eggs into a nonstick skillet that has been heated to medium heat.

When the eggs are set, add chopped vegetables to one side of the omelet.

After folding the omelet's other side over the veggies, cook it for one more minute to ensure it is thoroughly heated.

Accompany with a piece of whole grain toast for a high-fiber, blood-sugar-stabilizing breakfast.

2. Greek Yogurt with Berries and Almonds:

Ingredients:

1/2 cup plain Greek yogurt

1/4 cup mixed berries (such as strawberries, blueberries, and raspberries)

1 tablespoon sliced almonds

Instructions:

Spoon Greek yogurt into a bowl and top with mixed berries and sliced almonds.

Enjoy this protein-rich breakfast that provides a combination of fiber, vitamins, minerals, and healthy fats to support stable blood sugar levels.

3. Chia Seed Pudding with Fresh Fruit:

Ingredients:
2 tablespoons chia seeds
1/2 cup unsweetened almond milk
1/2 cup sliced fresh fruit (such as kiwi, pineapple, and mango).

Instructions:
Mix the almond milk and chia seeds in a jar or other container. Mix thoroughly to blend.
Cover and chill until the mixture thickens and takes on the consistency of pudding, which should take at least two hours or overnight.
For a low-GI, high-fiber, and antioxidant-rich breakfast option, serve chilled with sliced fresh fruit.

4. Quinoa Breakfast Bowl with Nuts and Cinnamon:

Ingredients:
Half a cup of cooked quinoa
One tablespoon of finely chopped nuts, like pecans, walnuts, or almonds
A dash of cinnamon.

Instructions:

In a bowl, combine cooked quinoa with chopped nuts and a sprinkle of cinnamon.

Mix well and enjoy this fiber-rich breakfast that provides sustained energy and stabilizes blood sugar levels throughout the morning.

5. Smoked Salmon and Avocado Toast on Rye Bread:

Ingredients:

1 slice rye bread, toasted

1/4 ripe avocado, mashed

2 ounces smoked salmon

Instructions:

Spread mashed avocado evenly over the toasted rye bread.

Top with smoked salmon slices for a protein-rich breakfast that's low in carbohydrates and has minimal impact on blood sugar levels.

6. Green Smoothie with Protein Powder:

Ingredients:
Handful of spinach or kale
1/2 banana
1 scoop of unsweetened protein powder (such as
pea protein or whey protein isolate)
1 cup unsweetened almond milk
Instructions:
Blend spinach or kale, banana, protein powder, and
almond milk until smooth and creamy.
Enjoy this nutrient-packed smoothie that's low in
sugar and high in protein, fiber, vitamins, and
minerals.

7. Egg and Veggie Breakfast Burrito with Whole Grain Tortilla:

Ingredients:
1 whole grain tortilla
2 scrambled eggs
Handful of sautéed vegetables (such as bell peppers,
onions, and zucchini).

Instructions:
Fill a whole grain tortilla with scrambled eggs and sautéed vegetables.
Roll up the tortilla and enjoy this savory breakfast option that's low in carbohydrates and high in protein and fiber.

You can enhance overall health and well-being, stabilize blood sugar levels, and improve insulin sensitivity by including these low-glycemic index breakfast ideas in your PCOS diet. To find options that fit your dietary requirements and taste preferences, try experimenting with different ingredients and flavor combinations.

CHAPTER FIVE

Lunch and Dinner Recipes

Here are some specific lunch and dinner recipes suitable for a PCOS diet:

Lunch Recipes:

Quinoa Salad with Chickpeas and Veggies:
Quinoa is a gluten-free whole grain rich in fiber, protein, and essential nutrients. It has a low glycemic index, which helps regulate blood sugar levels, making it ideal for PCOS management. Chickpeas are a good source of plant-based protein and fiber, promoting satiety and aiding in blood sugar control.

Adding a variety of colorful veggies like cucumbers, cherry tomatoes, and spinach increases the nutrient content and provides antioxidants, vitamins, and minerals essential for overall health. Dressing the salad with a vinaigrette made from olive oil, lemon juice, and herbs adds flavor and healthy fats, which are beneficial for hormone regulation in PCOS.

Grilled Chicken and Avocado Wrap:
Grilled chicken breast is a lean source of protein,
essential for muscle repair and hormone balance.
Avocado is rich in monounsaturated fats, which
help reduce inflammation and improve insulin
sensitivity.
Whole-grain tortillas provide complex
carbohydrates and fiber, which are digested slowly,
preventing blood sugar spikes.
Adding lettuce and shredded carrots increases the
fiber content and adds crunch, while Greek yogurt
or hummus provides additional protein and
creaminess without excess sugar or unhealthy fats.

Salmon and Quinoa Stuffed Bell Peppers:
Salmon is a fatty fish rich in omega-3 fatty acids,
which have anti-inflammatory properties and help
regulate hormones in PCOS.
Quinoa is a gluten-free grain high in protein and
fiber, promoting satiety and aiding in blood sugar
control.
Bell peppers are low in calories and high in
vitamins C and A, which support immune function
and skin health.

This dish is nutrient-dense, providing essential nutrients while being low in refined carbohydrates and processed ingredients, making it suitable for a PCOS diet.

Turkey and Vegetable Stir-Fry:
Lean ground turkey is a good source of protein and contains less saturated fat compared to red meat, making it heart-healthy and suitable for PCOS. Colorful vegetables like bell peppers, broccoli, and snap peas are rich in vitamins, minerals, and antioxidants, which help reduce inflammation and regulate hormones.
Ginger and garlic add flavor and have anti-inflammatory properties, while low-sodium soy sauce adds umami without excess sodium.
Serving the stir-fry over brown rice or cauliflower rice provides fiber and complex carbohydrates, promoting satiety and stable blood sugar levels.

Baked Cod with Roasted Vegetables:
Cod is a lean source of protein and a good source of vitamins B12 and B6, which are important for energy metabolism and hormone regulation.

Roasted vegetables like zucchini, bell peppers, and cherry tomatoes are rich in antioxidants and fiber, supporting gut health and hormone balance.
Baking the cod and vegetables with lemon juice, olive oil, and herbs adds flavor without excess calories or unhealthy fats, making it a nutritious and satisfying meal for PCOS management.

Dinner Recipes:

Vegetable and Lentil Curry:
Lentils are a plant-based source of protein and fiber, which help stabilize blood sugar levels and promote satiety.
Vegetables like cauliflower, carrots, and spinach are high in vitamins, minerals, and antioxidants, which support overall health and hormone balance.
Coconut milk adds creaminess and healthy fats, while curry powder and spices like turmeric and cumin provide flavor and anti-inflammatory benefits.
This dish is rich in plant-based nutrients and low in processed ingredients, making it suitable for a PCOS diet.

Turkey Meatballs with Zucchini Noodles:
Turkey meatballs are a lean source of protein and
contain less saturated fat compared to beef or pork,
making them heart-healthy and suitable for PCOS.
Zucchini noodles are low in calories and
carbohydrates and high in fiber, promoting satiety
and stable blood sugar levels.
Baking the meatballs and serving them with
marinara sauce made from tomatoes and herbs adds
flavor and nutrients without excess sugar or
unhealthy fats.
This dish is low in refined carbohydrates and
processed ingredients, making it a nutritious and
satisfying option for PCOS management.

Chickpea and Spinach Stuffed Sweet Potatoes:
Sweet potatoes are a nutrient-dense source of
complex carbohydrates, vitamins, and minerals,
which help regulate blood sugar levels and support
hormone balance.
Chickpeas are a plant-based source of protein and
fiber, which promote satiety and aid in blood sugar
control.

Spinach is rich in iron and folate, important nutrients for women with PCOS, and adds flavor and color to the dish.

This dish is rich in plant-based nutrients and low in processed ingredients, making it a healthy and satisfying option for PCOS management.

Mediterranean Chicken and Vegetable Skewers:
Chicken breast is a lean source of protein and contains essential amino acids necessary for muscle repair and hormone balance.

Mediterranean vegetables like cherry tomatoes, bell peppers, and onions are rich in antioxidants and vitamins, which support overall health and hormone regulation.

Skewering the chicken and vegetables and grilling them with olive oil and herbs adds flavor and healthy fats, making it a nutritious and satisfying meal for PCOS management.

Serving the skewers with a side of Greek yogurt mixed with herbs and lemon juice provides additional protein and creaminess without excess sugar or unhealthy fats.

Spinach and Feta Stuffed Chicken Breast:
Chicken breast is a lean source of protein and contains less saturated fat compared to red meat, making it heart-healthy and suitable for PCOS. Spinach is rich in iron and folate, important nutrients for women with PCOS, and adds flavor and color to the dish.
Feta cheese adds creaminess and flavor without excess calories or unhealthy fats, while also providing calcium and protein.
Baking the stuffed chicken breast with lemon juice, olive oil, and herbs adds flavor without excess calories or unhealthy fats, making it a nutritious and satisfying option for PCOS management.

These lunch and dinner recipes are designed to be balanced and nutritious, providing essential nutrients while supporting hormone balance and blood sugar control in women with PCOS. Incorporating a variety of whole foods, lean proteins, healthy fats, and colorful vegetables into meals can help manage symptoms and improve overall health and well-being.

Balanced meals for lunch and dinner

Balanced meals are essential for managing PCOS (Polycystic Ovary Syndrome) as they help regulate blood sugar levels, support hormone balance, and maintain a healthy weight. Here's a comprehensive guide on balanced meals for lunch and dinner in a PCOS diet:

Lunch:

Protein Source:
Incorporate lean protein sources such as grilled chicken breast, turkey, tofu, tempeh, or legumes like lentils and chickpeas.
Protein helps stabilize blood sugar levels, promotes satiety, and supports muscle repair and hormone balance.

Healthy Fats:
Include sources of healthy fats like avocado, nuts, seeds, and olive oil.
Healthy fats aid in hormone production and absorption of fat-soluble vitamins, and they help keep you feeling full and satisfied.

Complex Carbohydrates:

Option for complex carbohydrates with a low
glycemic index, such as quinoa, brown rice, sweet
potatoes, or whole-grain bread and pasta.
Complex carbs are digested more slowly,
preventing blood sugar spikes and providing
sustained energy.

Fiber-Rich Vegetables:
Fill half of your plate with non-starchy vegetables
like leafy greens, broccoli, cauliflower, bell
peppers, and zucchini.
Vegetables are high in fiber, vitamins, and minerals,
promoting digestion, reducing inflammation, and
supporting hormone balance.

Hydration:
Stay hydrated by drinking water or herbal teas
throughout the day.
Adequate hydration supports metabolic function,
aids digestion, and helps flush out toxins from the
body.

Dinner:

Lean Protein:
Choose lean protein sources for dinner, such as fish
(salmon, cod), poultry (chicken, turkey), lean cuts
of beef or pork, or plant-based proteins like tofu and
legumes.
Protein-rich foods provide amino acids necessary
for hormone synthesis and repair of tissues.

Healthy Fats:
Include sources of healthy fats like fatty fish
(salmon, mackerel), olive oil, avocado, nuts, and
seeds.
Omega-3 fatty acids found in fish and plant-based
fats support hormone regulation and reduce
inflammation associated with PCOS.

Colorful Vegetables:
Fill your plate with a variety of colorful vegetables
such as spinach, kale, tomatoes, carrots, and
Brussels sprouts.
Colorful veggies are rich in antioxidants, vitamins,
and minerals that support overall health and
hormone balance.

Whole Grains:

Incorporate whole grains such as quinoa, brown rice, barley, or whole-grain pasta into your dinner. Whole grains provide fiber, B vitamins, and minerals, promoting satiety and stable blood sugar levels.

Balanced Portions:
Take note of portion sizes to prevent overindulging and encourage healthy weight management.
50% non-starchy veggies, 25% lean protein, and 25% whole grains or healthy fats should make up a balanced plate.

Tips for Creating Balanced Meals:

Meal Planning: Arrange your meals in advance to guarantee that they are wholesome and well-balanced.

Incorporate Variety: Include a variety of foods from all food groups to ensure you're getting a wide range of nutrients.

Limit Processed Foods: Minimize intake of processed foods, sugary snacks, and refined carbohydrates, which can disrupt hormone balance and insulin sensitivity.

Listen to Your Body: Pay attention to hunger and fullness cues, and eat until you're satisfied, but not overly full.

Stay Consistent: Aim to eat balanced meals consistently throughout the day to maintain stable energy levels and support overall health.

You can enhance hormone balance, better manage PCOS symptoms, and enhance your general health and well-being by including balanced meals in your lunch and dinner routine.

One-pot meals for easy cleanup

One-pot meals are perfect for those following a PCOS diet because they're convenient, require minimal cleanup, and can be packed with nutritious ingredients. Here's a comprehensive explanation of one-pot meals tailored for the PCOS diet:

Benefits of One-Pot Meals for PCOS Diet:

Convenience: One-pot meals are simple to prepare and require minimal cooking skills. They're perfect for busy individuals managing PCOS symptoms who need quick and easy meal options.

Minimal Cleanup: With only one pot or pan used for cooking, cleanup is a breeze. This is especially helpful for those with PCOS who may experience fatigue or lack of energy and motivation to clean up after cooking.

Balanced Nutrition: One-pot meals can be packed with a variety of nutrient-dense ingredients, including lean proteins, whole grains, healthy fats, and plenty of vegetables, all of which are important components of a PCOS-friendly diet.

Controlled Portions: By cooking everything together in one pot, it's easier to control portion sizes and ensure a balanced meal, which is important for managing weight and blood sugar levels in individuals with PCOS.

Example One-Pot Meals for PCOS Diet:

Quinoa and Vegetable Stir-Fry:
Cook quinoa in a pot according to package instructions.
In the same pot, stir-fry diced vegetables such as bell peppers, broccoli, carrots, and snap peas with a lean protein like tofu or chicken breast.
For flavor, add low-sodium soy sauce, ginger, and garlic.
Quinoa provides fiber and protein, while vegetables offer vitamins and minerals essential for hormone balance.

Lentil and Vegetable Soup:
In a large pot, sauté onions, garlic, and celery until soft.
Add dried lentils, diced tomatoes, vegetable broth, and a mix of chopped vegetables like carrots, spinach, and zucchini.

Season with herbs and spices like thyme, oregano, and bay leaves.
Simmer until lentils and vegetables are tender, creating a hearty and nutritious soup packed with fiber and plant-based protein.

Salmon and Asparagus Bake:
Place salmon filets and trimmed asparagus spears on a baking sheet lined with parchment paper.
Drizzle with olive oil and season with lemon juice, garlic, and herbs like dill or parsley.
Bake in the oven until salmon is cooked through and asparagus is tender.
Serve with a side of quinoa or brown rice for a complete and balanced meal rich in omega-3 fatty acids, protein, and fiber.

Mediterranean Chickpea Skillet:
In a large skillet, sauté onions, garlic, and diced bell peppers in olive oil until softened.
Add canned chickpeas, cherry tomatoes, and chopped spinach to the skillet.
Season with Mediterranean spices like oregano, basil, and paprika.

Cook until vegetables are tender and flavors are combined, creating a flavorful and satisfying meal rich in fiber, protein, and healthy fats.

Tips for One-Pot Meals:

Choose Nutrient-Dense Ingredients: Option for whole grains, lean proteins, healthy fats, and plenty of vegetables to ensure your one-pot meal is packed with essential nutrients.

Experiment with Flavors: Don't be afraid to get creative with herbs, spices, and seasonings to add flavor without excess salt or sugar.

Prep Ahead: Chop vegetables and portion out ingredients ahead of time to streamline the cooking process and make meal prep even easier.

Customize to Taste: Feel free to customize one-pot meals based on your preferences and dietary restrictions. Swap out ingredients or adjust seasonings as needed to suit your taste buds.

Protein-rich dishes to support hormone balance

Including high-protein foods in a PCOS diet is essential for maintaining blood sugar stability, controlling weight, and promoting hormone balance. Here are a few recipes full of protein that are suitable for people with PCOS:

Grilled Salmon with Quinoa and Steamed Broccoli:
Salmon is rich in omega-3 fatty acids, which have anti-inflammatory properties and support hormone regulation.
Quinoa provides a good source of protein and fiber, aiding in blood sugar control and promoting satiety. Steamed broccoli adds fiber, vitamins, and minerals, enhancing the nutritional profile of the meal.

Turkey and Vegetable Stir-Fry with Brown Rice:
Lean ground turkey serves as a high-protein base for this dish, supporting muscle health and hormone balance.
Colorful vegetables like bell peppers, carrots, and

snap peas provide additional fiber, vitamins, and antioxidants.
Brown rice is a complex carbohydrate that offers sustained energy and helps regulate blood sugar levels.

Greek Yogurt Parfait with Berries and Almonds:
Greek yogurt is packed with protein and probiotics, which support gut health and hormone balance.
Fresh berries add natural sweetness and antioxidants, while almonds provide healthy fats and additional protein.
This parfait is a satisfying and nutrient-dense snack or dessert option for individuals with PCOS.

Quinoa and Black Bean Salad with Avocado Dressing:
Quinoa and black beans combine to create a complete protein source, offering all essential amino acids necessary for hormone synthesis.
Avocado dressing made with avocado, lime juice, and cilantro adds healthy fats and creaminess to the salad.

This salad is rich in fiber, protein, and micronutrients, making it an ideal choice for a PCOS-friendly meal.

Egg and Vegetable Frittata with Spinach Salad:
Eggs are a versatile and affordable source of high-quality protein, essential for hormone regulation and muscle repair.
A vegetable frittata made with bell peppers, onions, and spinach adds fiber and vitamins to the meal.
A side salad of fresh spinach provides additional nutrients and fiber, promoting satiety and supporting digestive health.

Tofu and Vegetable Stir-Fry with Cauliflower Rice:
Tofu is a plant-based source of protein that also contains phytoestrogens, which may help regulate hormone levels in individuals with PCOS.
Stir-frying tofu with colorful vegetables like bell peppers, broccoli, and mushrooms creates a flavorful and nutritious dish.
Serving the stir-fry over cauliflower rice instead of traditional rice reduces carbohydrates and calories while increasing fiber content.

Chicken and Quinoa Soup with Kale:
Chicken breast is a lean source of protein that provides essential amino acids necessary for hormone synthesis and muscle repair.
Quinoa adds protein and fiber to the soup, making it a hearty and satisfying meal option.
Kale is rich in vitamins A, C, and K, as well as antioxidants, which support overall health and hormone balance.

Lentil and Vegetable Curry with Brown Rice:
Lentils are a plant-based source of protein and fiber, which promote satiety and aid in blood sugar control.
A vegetable curry made with lentils, tomatoes, onions, and spices provides a flavorful and nutrient-rich dish.
Serving the curry over brown rice adds complex carbohydrates and additional fiber, creating a balanced and satisfying meal.

Baked Chicken Thighs with Roasted Vegetables:
Chicken thighs are higher in fat than chicken breasts
but still provide a good source of protein, as well as
essential nutrients like iron and zinc.
Roasting vegetables like carrots, Brussels sprouts,
and sweet potatoes alongside the chicken adds fiber,
vitamins, and minerals to the meal.
This simple and flavorful dish is easy to prepare and
can be customized with your favorite herbs and
spices.

Salmon and Avocado Sushi Bowl:
Salmon is rich in omega-3 fatty acids, which
support hormone regulation and reduce
inflammation.
Avocado adds healthy fats and creaminess to the
sushi bowl, while also providing vitamins and
minerals.
Serve the salmon and avocado over a base of brown
rice or cauliflower rice, and add additional
vegetables like cucumber, carrots, and seaweed for
extra nutrients and fiber.

CHAPTER SIX

Snacks and Appetizers

Snacks and appetizers play a significant role in a PCOS (Polycystic Ovary Syndrome) diet, as they can help stabilize blood sugar levels, manage weight, and curb cravings. Here are some comprehensive ideas for snacks and appetizers suitable for individuals with PCOS:

Snacks:

Greek Yogurt with Berries and Almonds: Greek yogurt is high in protein and probiotics, which support gut health and hormone balance. Add fresh berries for natural sweetness and antioxidants, and top with almonds for healthy fats and additional protein.

Vegetable Sticks with Hummus:
Slice carrots, cucumber, bell peppers, and celery
into sticks for a crunchy and satisfying snack.
Pair with hummus for a protein-rich dip that also
provides healthy fats and fiber.

Hard-Boiled Eggs:
Hard-boiled eggs are a convenient and portable
snack packed with protein, essential for hormone
regulation and satiety.
For added taste, add a small pinch of salt and
pepper.

Avocado Toast on Whole Grain Bread:
Mash avocado onto whole grain toast for a creamy
and nutritious snack.
Avocado provides healthy fats, while whole grain
bread offers fiber and complex carbohydrates.

Trail Mix with Nuts and Dried Fruit:
Create a homemade trail mix with a variety of nuts
(such as almonds, walnuts, and cashews) and dried
fruit (like apricots, raisins, and cranberries).
Nuts provide protein and healthy fats, while dried
fruit adds natural sweetness and fiber.

Appetizers:

Caprese Salad Skewers:
Skewer cherry tomatoes, fresh mozzarella balls, and basil leaves onto toothpicks for a colorful and refreshing appetizer.
Drizzle with balsamic glaze and sprinkle with sea salt for added flavor.

Spinach and Feta Stuffed Mushrooms:
Remove the stems from button mushrooms and fill with a mixture of sautéed spinach, garlic, and crumbled feta cheese.
Bake until the filling is heated through and the mushrooms are soft.

Cucumber Cups with Tuna Salad:
To make cups, slice cucumbers into thick rounds and hollow out the centers.
Spoon canned tuna, Greek yogurt, diced celery, and lemon juice into each cucumber cup.

Smoked Salmon and Cucumber Bites:
Cut English cucumber into thick slices and top with smoked salmon.
Garnish with a dollop of Greek yogurt and fresh dill for a flavorful and elegant appetizer.

Stuffed Bell Peppers with Quinoa and Black Beans:
Halve bell peppers and remove seeds and membranes.
Fill each pepper half with a mixture of cooked quinoa, black beans, diced tomatoes, corn, and spices like cumin and chili powder.
Bake until the peppers are soft and the filling is thoroughly heated.

Tips for Snacks and Appetizers in a PCOS Diet:

Portion Control: Pay attention to portion sizes to avoid overeating, especially with calorie-dense snacks like nuts and dried fruit.

Balance Macronutrients: Aim to include a combination of protein, healthy fats, and complex carbohydrates in your snacks and appetizers to support blood sugar control and satiety.

Choose Whole Foods: Option for whole, minimally processed ingredients whenever possible to maximize nutrient intake and minimize added sugars and unhealthy fats.

Keep Yourself Hydrated: A lot of water should be consumed throughout the day because sometimes hunger is confused with thirst. Water or herbal tea are better options than sugar-filled drinks.

Plan Ahead: Prepare snacks and appetizers in advance to have healthy options readily available when hunger strikes, reducing the temptation to reach for less nutritious choices.

Healthy snack options to keep you satisfied between meals

Choosing healthy snacks is essential for individuals following a PCOS (Polycystic Ovary Syndrome) diet, as it helps stabilize blood sugar levels, manage weight, and prevent overeating during meals. Here are some comprehensive options for healthy snacks to keep you satisfied between meals:

1. Greek Yogurt with Berries and Almonds:
Greek yogurt is high in protein and probiotics, which support gut health and hormone balance. Add fresh berries like strawberries, blueberries, or raspberries for natural sweetness and antioxidants. Sprinkle with almonds or walnuts for healthy fats and additional protein, helping to keep you feeling full and satisfied.

2. Vegetable Sticks with Hummus:
Slice carrots, cucumber, bell peppers, and celery into sticks for a crunchy and satisfying snack. Pair with hummus, which is made from chickpeas and tahini, providing protein, fiber, and healthy fats.

Hummus also contains various vitamins and minerals, including iron and magnesium, which are beneficial for individuals with PCOS.

3. Hard-Boiled Eggs:
Hard-boiled eggs are a convenient and portable snack packed with high-quality protein.
Protein helps stabilize blood sugar levels and promotes satiety, making hard-boiled eggs an excellent option for managing hunger between meals.
Enjoy them plain or sprinkle with a pinch of salt and pepper for added flavor.

4. Avocado Toast on Whole Grain Bread:
Mash avocado onto whole grain toast for a creamy and nutritious snack.
Avocado is rich in healthy fats, particularly monounsaturated fats, which have been shown to improve insulin sensitivity in individuals with PCOS.
Whole grain bread provides complex carbohydrates and fiber, promoting stable energy levels and supporting digestive health.

5. Trail Mix with Nuts and Dried Fruit:
Create a homemade trail mix by combining a variety of nuts such as almonds, walnuts, and cashews with dried fruits like apricots, raisins, and cranberries.
Nuts are a good source of protein, healthy fats, and fiber, while dried fruits add natural sweetness and additional fiber.
Because nuts and dried fruits are high in calories, watch how much you eat.

6. Cottage Cheese with Pineapple:
Cottage cheese is rich in protein and low in carbohydrates, making it an excellent snack option for individuals with PCOS.
Pair with fresh pineapple chunks for a sweet and tangy flavor combination.
Pineapple contains bromelain, an enzyme that may help reduce inflammation and support digestion.

7. Edamame:
Edamame, also known as young soybeans, are a healthy snack that is high in fiber, protein, and a variety of vitamins and minerals.

Enjoy them steamed and sprinkled with a pinch of
sea salt for a satisfying and crunchy snack.
Edamame is also a good source of phytoestrogens,
which may help balance hormone levels in
individuals with PCOS.

8. Apple Slices with Almond Butter:
Slice a fresh apple and spread almond butter on
each slice for a delicious and nutritious snack.
Apples are high in fiber and antioxidants, while
almond butter provides protein and healthy fats.
This combination offers a satisfying blend of sweet
and savory flavors, keeping you full and energized
between meals.

9. Roasted Chickpeas:
Drain and rinse canned chickpeas, then toss with
olive oil and your favorite seasonings like garlic
powder, paprika, and cumin.
Roast in the oven until crispy for a crunchy and
flavorful snack.
Chickpeas are rich in protein and fiber, making
them an excellent choice for promoting satiety and
supporting digestive health.

10. **Veggie and Hummus Wrap:**
Spread hummus onto a whole grain tortilla and fill
with sliced vegetables such as cucumber, bell
peppers, carrots, and spinach.
Roll up the tortilla and slice into bite-sized pieces
for a convenient and satisfying snack.
This snack option provides a good balance of
protein, fiber, and complex carbohydrates, helping
to keep you full and satisfied until your next meal.

Tips for Healthy Snacking on a PCOS Diet:

Portion Control: Be mindful of portion sizes,
especially with calorie-dense foods like nuts and
dried fruits.

Stay Hydrated: To stay hydrated and avoid
confusing thirst for hunger, drink a lot of water
throughout the day.

Plan Ahead: Prepare snacks in advance and portion
them into single servings to avoid reaching for less
healthy options when hunger strikes.

Listen to Your Body: Pay attention to hunger and
fullness cues, and eat when you're hungry rather
than out of boredom or habit.

Portable snack ideas for on-the-go lifestyles

Having portable snack options is crucial for people with hectic schedules who are on a PCOS (Polycystic Ovary Syndrome) diet to maintain good eating habits when they're on the go. Here are a few thorough suggestions for healthy, portable snacks that fit well with a PCOS diet:

1. **Protein Bars:**

Look for protein bars made with natural ingredients and minimal added sugars.
Choose bars with a good balance of protein, healthy fats, and fiber to keep you feeling full and satisfied. Opt for bars with at least 10 grams of protein and less than 10 grams of sugar per serving.

2. **String Cheese or Cheese Sticks:**

String cheese or individually wrapped cheese sticks are convenient and portable sources of protein and calcium.
Pair with whole grain crackers or a piece of fruit for a balanced snack option.

3. **Nut Butter Packets:**

Single-serve packets of almond butter, peanut butter, or other nut butters are portable and mess-free.
Spread nut butter on whole grain crackers, apple slices, or celery sticks for a quick and satisfying snack.

4. **Greek Yogurt Cups:**

Individual containers of Greek yogurt are convenient for on-the-go snacking.
Look for Greek yogurt with no added sugars and a high protein content to support hormone balance and satiety.

5. **Trail Mix:**

Prepare your own trail mix with a mix of nuts, seeds, and dried fruit.
Be mindful of portion sizes and choose unsweetened dried fruit to minimize added sugars.

6. Hard-Boiled Eggs:

Hard-boiled eggs are portable and packed with protein, making them an ideal snack option for busy days.
Season with a sprinkle of salt and pepper or your favorite spices for extra flavor.

7. Veggie Sticks with Hummus:

Pre-cut vegetables like carrots, celery, cucumber, and bell peppers are convenient for snacking on the go.
Pair with single-serve containers of hummus for a satisfying and nutritious snack.

8. Rice Cakes with Avocado:

Pack rice cakes and individual packets of mashed avocado for a quick and easy snack.
Top rice cakes with avocado and a sprinkle of sea salt for a delicious and satisfying treat.

9. Tuna or Chicken Salad Packets:

Look for single-serve packets of tuna or chicken salad made with simple, wholesome ingredients.
Enjoy whole grain crackers, rice cakes, or wrapped in lettuce leaves for a protein-rich snack.

10. **Fresh Fruit:**
Apples, bananas, oranges, and grapes are
convenient and portable options for on-the-go
snacking.
Pair with a handful of nuts or a piece of string
cheese for a balanced snack that combines protein,
healthy fats, and fiber.

Tips for Portable Snacking on a PCOS Diet:

Plan Ahead: Prepare snacks in advance and portion
them into single servings to grab and go when
you're on the move.

Choose Nutrient-Dense Options: Select snacks
that provide a good balance of protein, healthy fats,
and fiber to keep you feeling satisfied and
energized.

Stay Hydrated: Bring a reusable water bottle with
you to stay hydrated throughout the day, as
dehydration can sometimes be mistaken for hunger.

Be Mindful of Portions: Pay attention to portion sizes, especially with calorie-dense snacks like nuts and nut butter, to avoid overeating.

Listen to Your Body: Eat when you're hungry and stop when you're satisfied, and choose snacks that support your overall health and well-being.

Appetizers suitable for parties and gatherings

When hosting or attending parties and gatherings while following a PCOS (Polycystic Ovary Syndrome) diet, it's important to have appetizer options that are both delicious and supportive of your dietary needs. Here are some comprehensive ideas for appetizers suitable for parties and gatherings on a PCOS diet:

1. **Veggie Platter with Greek Yogurt Dip:**
Arrange a variety of colorful vegetables such as carrots, celery, bell peppers, cucumber, and cherry tomatoes on a platter.
Serve with a creamy Greek yogurt dip flavored with herbs and spices like dill, garlic, and lemon juice. Greek yogurt provides protein and probiotics, while vegetables offer fiber, vitamins, and minerals.

2. **Caprese Skewers:**
Skewer cherry tomatoes, fresh mozzarella balls, and basil leaves onto toothpicks for a classic and elegant appetizer.
Drizzle with balsamic glaze and sprinkle with sea salt for added flavor.
This appetizer provides protein, calcium, and antioxidants, making it a nutritious and crowd-pleasing option.

3. **Smoked Salmon Cucumber Bites:**
Slice English cucumber into rounds and top each with a small piece of smoked salmon.
Garnish with a dollop of Greek yogurt or cream cheese and fresh dill or chives.
Smoked salmon is rich in omega-3 fatty acids, while cucumber adds hydration and crunch.

4. **Stuffed Mushrooms with Spinach and Feta:**
Remove stems from button mushrooms and fill each cap with a mixture of sautéed spinach, garlic, and crumbled feta cheese.
Bake until the filling is heated through and the mushrooms are soft.

Mushrooms are low in calories and rich in vitamins and minerals, while spinach provides iron and feta adds flavor and creaminess.

5. Mini Quinoa and Black Bean Stuffed Peppers:
Halve mini bell peppers and remove seeds and membranes.
Fill each pepper half with a mixture of cooked quinoa, black beans, diced tomatoes, corn, and spices like cumin and chili powder.
Bake until the peppers are soft and the filling is thoroughly heated.
Bell peppers contribute color and vitamins, while black beans and quinoa offer protein and fiber.

6. Tuna Cucumber Cups:
Slice English cucumber into thick rounds and hollow out the centers to create cups.
Fill each cucumber cup with a mixture of canned tuna, Greek yogurt, diced celery, and lemon juice.
Top with a sprinkle of paprika or chopped parsley for garnish.
Tuna provides protein and omega-3 fatty acids, while cucumber adds hydration and crunch.

7. Chicken Lettuce Wraps:
Cook ground chicken with minced garlic, ginger,
and diced vegetables like water chestnuts, carrots,
and bell peppers.
Spoon chicken mixture into large lettuce leaves,
such as butter or romaine lettuce.
Drizzle with a homemade Asian-inspired sauce
made from soy sauce, sesame oil, and rice vinegar.
These lettuce wraps are low in carbohydrates and
can be customized with your favorite ingredients.

8. Deviled Eggs with Avocado:
Hard-boil eggs and cut in half lengthwise. Remove
yolks and mash with ripe avocado, Dijon mustard,
and a splash of lemon juice.
Spoon avocado mixture back into egg whites and
garnish with paprika or fresh herbs.
Eggs are a good source of protein and healthy fats,
while avocado adds creaminess and additional
nutrients.

9. Coconut Shrimp with Mango Salsa:
Coat shrimp in shredded coconut and bake until golden and crispy.
Serve with a homemade mango salsa made from diced mango, red onion, cilantro, lime juice, and jalapeño.
Shrimp provides protein and healthy fats, while mango salsa adds sweetness and a burst of flavor.

10. Mediterranean Mezze Platter:
Arrange a variety of Mediterranean-inspired appetizers on a platter, such as olives, hummus, feta cheese, grape leaves, and whole grain crackers or pita bread.
Add sliced vegetables like cucumbers, cherry tomatoes, and bell peppers for extra crunch and freshness.
This customizable platter offers a mix of protein, healthy fats, and fiber-rich carbohydrates, making it suitable for a PCOS diet.

Tips for PCOS-Friendly Appetizers:

Choose Whole Foods: Option for whole, minimally processed ingredients whenever possible to maximize nutrient intake and minimize added sugars and unhealthy fats.

Focus on Protein and Fiber: Incorporate protein-rich foods like lean meats, fish, eggs, legumes, and Greek yogurt, as well as fiber-rich vegetables and whole grains, to support blood sugar control and satiety.

Use Healthy Fats: Include sources of healthy fats such as avocado, nuts, seeds, and olive oil to promote hormone balance and support overall health.

Mind Your Portions: Be mindful of portion sizes, especially with calorie-dense foods like nuts, cheese, and dips, to avoid overeating.

Stay Hydrated: Offer hydrating options like infused water, sparkling water, or herbal tea alongside appetizers to help guests stay hydrated throughout the event.

You can provide tasty and healthy options that everyone will appreciate at your party or get-together while also supporting your dietary goals and advancing general health and well-being by serving these PCOS-friendly appetizers.

CHAPTER SEVEN

Desserts and Treats

When it comes to desserts and treats for individuals following a PCOS (Polycystic Ovary Syndrome) diet, it's important to focus on options that are not only delicious but also supportive of hormone balance and overall health. Here are some comprehensive ideas for desserts and treats suitable for a PCOS diet:

1. **Fruit Salad with Greek Yogurt:**
In a bowl, mix together various fresh fruits like mango, pineapple, kiwi, and berries.
For extra protein and creaminess, top with a dollop of Greek yogurt and serve.
Fruits add natural sweetness and vitamins, and Greek yogurt offers probiotics and protein.

2. **Dark Chocolate Covered Almonds:**
Place raw almonds on a baking sheet covered with parchment paper after dipping them in melted dark chocolate.

Before serving, let the chocolate cool in the fridge and solidify.

Almonds offer protein and healthy fats, while dark chocolate has antioxidants and may improve insulin sensitivity.

3. **Chia Seed Pudding:**

In a bowl or jar, combine chia seeds with unsweetened almond or coconut milk.

Stir in flavorings (like vanilla extract or cocoa powder) and a natural sweetener (like stevia or honey).

Put the mixture in the fridge for several hours or even overnight to thicken.

Because chia seeds are rich in omega-3 fatty acids and fiber, this pudding is a filling and healthy dessert choice.

4. **Baked Apples with Cinnamon and Walnuts:**

After coring the apples, put them in a baking dish.

Place a mixture of chopped walnuts, cinnamon, and either honey or maple syrup inside each apple.

Bake until the filling is bubbling and the apples are soft.

Walnuts provide crunch and healthy fats, and apples are rich in fiber and antioxidants.

5. Frozen Yogurt Bark:
On a baking sheet covered with parchment paper, spread the Greek yogurt.
Add sliced almonds, fresh berries, and a drizzle of melted dark chocolate or honey on top.
Break into pieces to serve after freezing until solid.
Berries contribute sweetness and antioxidants, and Greek yogurt supplies both protein and probiotics.

6. Banana Oat Cookies:
Ripe bananas should be mashed and combined with rolled oats, cinnamon, and a small amount of chopped nuts or dark chocolate chips.
Spoonfuls of the mixture should be placed onto a baking sheet, then baked until solid and golden.
These cookies have fiber, potassium, and healthy carbohydrates in addition to being naturally sweetened with bananas.

7. Avocado Chocolate Mousse:
Blend together ripe avocado, cocoa powder, a small amount of almond milk, and a natural sweetener such as dates or maple syrup.
Refrigerate until it becomes creamy and thick.

Cocoa powder offers antioxidants and a deep chocolate flavor, while avocado adds creaminess and healthy fats.

8. Coconut Flour Pancakes:
Mix coconut flour with eggs, almond milk, and a natural sweetener like stevia or honey.
Cook pancakes on a griddle until golden and fluffy.
Coconut flour is lower in carbohydrates and higher in fiber than traditional flour, making these pancakes a PCOS-friendly option.

9. Berry Crisp with Almond Flour Topping:
Toss mixed berries with a squeeze of lemon juice and a natural sweetener like honey or maple syrup.
Top with a mixture of almond flour, chopped nuts, cinnamon, and a drizzle of melted coconut oil or butter.
Bake until bubbly and golden brown.
Berries are rich in antioxidants and fiber, while almond flour adds a nutty flavor and healthy fats.

10. **Pumpkin Spice Energy Bites:**
Combine rolled oats, pumpkin puree, almond butter,
pumpkin pie spice, and a natural sweetener like
maple syrup or dates in a food processor.
Roll mixture into bite-sized balls and coat with
shredded coconut or chopped nuts if desired.
Chill in the refrigerator until firm.
These energy bites are packed with fiber, protein,
and healthy fats, making them a satisfying and
nutritious treat.

Tips for PCOS-Friendly Desserts and Treats:

Use Natural Sweeteners: Option for natural
sweeteners like honey, maple syrup, stevia, or dates
to sweeten desserts without causing spikes in blood
sugar levels.

Incorporate Healthy Fats: Include sources of
healthy fats such as nuts, seeds, avocado, and
coconut oil to promote satiety and support hormone
balance.

Focus on Whole Foods: Choose desserts made with whole, minimally processed ingredients to maximize nutrient intake and minimize added sugars and unhealthy fats.

Watch Portion Sizes: Be mindful of portion sizes to avoid overindulging, especially with calorie-dense treats like nuts, seeds, and dark chocolate.

Experiment with Flavor: Get creative with flavorings like cinnamon, vanilla extract, cocoa powder, and citrus zest to add depth and complexity to your desserts.

These PCOS-friendly sweets and treats will help you manage weight, support hormone balance, and sate your sweet tooth while also enhancing your general health and well-being.

Guilt-free dessert options for satisfying cravings

Finding guilt-free dessert options that satisfy cravings while adhering to a PCOS (Polycystic Ovary Syndrome) diet can be challenging, but it's definitely possible with the right approach. Here are some comprehensive ideas for guilt-free dessert options tailored for individuals with PCOS:

1. Berry Parfait with Greek Yogurt:
Layer mixed berries (such as strawberries, blueberries, and raspberries) with plain Greek yogurt in a glass.
Add a sprinkle of granola or chopped nuts for crunch and texture.
Greek yogurt provides protein and probiotics, while berries offer natural sweetness and antioxidants.

2. Frozen Banana Bites:
Slice ripe bananas into rounds and place them on a baking sheet lined with parchment paper.

Spread almond butter or peanut butter on half of the banana rounds and top with the remaining rounds to create sandwiches.

Freeze until firm, then dip in melted dark chocolate and sprinkle with chopped nuts or shredded coconut if desired.
Bananas provide natural sweetness and potassium, while nut butter adds protein and healthy fats.

3. Coconut Chia Seed Pudding:
In a bowl or jar, combine chia seeds and unsweetened coconut milk.
Stir in a small amount of vanilla extract and a natural sweetener, such as stevia or honey.
Put the mixture in the fridge for several hours or even overnight to thicken.
For extra taste and texture, sprinkle fresh fruit or toasted coconut flakes on top.
Due to the high fiber and omega-3 fatty acid content of chia seeds, this pudding is a filling and guilt-free dessert choice.

4. Chocolate Avocado Mousse:

Blend ripe avocado with cocoa powder, a natural
sweetener like maple syrup or dates, and a splash of
almond milk until smooth and creamy.
Chill in the refrigerator until thickened.

Avocado adds creaminess and healthy fats, while
cocoa powder provides antioxidants and a rich
chocolate flavor.
Serve topped with sliced strawberries or raspberries
for extra sweetness.

5. Baked Apple Crisp:

After coring the apples, put them in a baking dish.
Place a mixture of chopped nuts, cinnamon, and
rolled oats inside each apple, then top with a drizzle
of honey or maple syrup.
Bake until the topping is crisp and golden and the
apples are soft.
Oats and nuts add crunch and heart-healthy fats,
while apples are high in antioxidants and fiber.
For extra protein, top with a drizzle of almond
butter or a dollop of Greek yogurt.

6. Lemon Coconut Energy Balls:

Combine rolled oats, shredded coconut, almond
flour, lemon zest, a natural sweetener like honey or

dates, and a splash of lemon juice in a food
processor.
Pulse until mixture comes together, then roll into
bite-sized balls.
Chill in the refrigerator until firm.

These energy balls are packed with fiber, protein,
and healthy fats, making them a satisfying and
guilt-free snack or dessert option.

7. Greek Yogurt Bark with Berries:

On a baking sheet covered with parchment paper,
spread out the plain Greek yogurt.
Add chopped nuts, mixed berries, and a drizzle of
maple syrup or honey on top.
Break into pieces to serve after freezing until solid.
Berries offer natural sweetness and antioxidants,
and Greek yogurt supplies both protein and
probiotics.

8. Pumpkin Spice Oatmeal Cookies:

Mix rolled oats with canned pumpkin puree,
cinnamon, nutmeg, and a natural sweetener like
maple syrup or stevia.
Drop spoonfuls of the mixture onto a baking sheet
lined with parchment paper and flatten slightly.

Bake until golden and firm.
These cookies are naturally sweetened with
pumpkin and provide fiber, vitamins, and minerals.

9. **Almond Flour Brownies:**
Combine almond flour with cocoa powder, a natural
sweetener like coconut sugar or honey, eggs, and
melted coconut oil.
Stir in dark chocolate chips or chopped nuts if
desired.
Bake in a square baking pan until set and fudgy.
Almond flour is lower in carbohydrates and higher
in protein and healthy fats than traditional flour,
making these brownies a guilt-free indulgence.

10. **Mint Chocolate Chip Smoothie Bowl:**
Blend frozen bananas with fresh spinach, mint
leaves, unsweetened almond milk, and a scoop of
protein powder until smooth and creamy.
Pour into a bowl and top with dark chocolate chips
or cacao nibs for crunch.
Enjoy with a spoon for a refreshing and guilt-free
dessert option.

Spinach adds nutrients and fiber, while bananas provide natural sweetness and potassium.

Tips for Guilt-Free Desserts on a PCOS Diet:

Focus on Whole Foods: Choose desserts made with whole, minimally processed ingredients to maximize nutrient intake and minimize added sugars and unhealthy fats.

Use Natural Sweeteners: Option for natural sweeteners like honey, maple syrup, stevia, or dates to sweeten desserts without causing spikes in blood sugar levels.

Incorporate Healthy Fats: Include sources of healthy fats such as nuts, seeds, avocado, and coconut oil to promote satiety and support hormone balance.

Watch Portion Sizes: Be mindful of portion sizes to avoid overindulging, especially with calorie-dense treats like nuts, seeds, and dark chocolate.

Get Creative with Flavor: Experiment with different flavor combinations and ingredients to keep desserts interesting and satisfying.

Sweet treats without spiking blood sugar levels

Finding sweet treats that don't spike blood sugar levels is crucial for individuals following a PCOS (Polycystic Ovary Syndrome) diet. Here are some comprehensive ideas for sweet treats that are low in added sugars and won't cause significant blood sugar spikes:

1. Fresh Fruit Salad:

Combine a variety of fresh fruits such as berries, melon, pineapple, and citrus segments in a bowl. Add a squeeze of lemon or lime juice and a sprinkle of cinnamon for extra flavor.

Fresh fruits provide natural sweetness and are rich in vitamins, minerals, and antioxidants.

2. **Yogurt Parfait with Nuts and Berries:**
Layer plain Greek yogurt with mixed berries and
chopped nuts in a glass or bowl.
Drizzle with a small amount of honey or maple
syrup if desired.
Greek yogurt is high in protein and probiotics,
while nuts add crunch and healthy fats.

3. **Baked Apples with Cinnamon:**
After coring the apples, put them in a baking dish.
After adding a cinnamon sprinkle, bake until soft.
Garnish with chopped nuts or a dollop of Greek
yogurt and serve warm.
Apples are a great source of antioxidants and fiber,
and cinnamon, without any added sugar, adds flavor
and warmth.

4. **Coconut Flour Pancakes:**
Mix coconut flour with eggs, almond milk, and a
natural sweetener like stevia or monk fruit
sweetener.
Cook pancakes on a griddle until golden and fluffy.
Coconut flour is lower in carbohydrates and higher
in fiber than traditional flour, making these
pancakes a PCOS-friendly option.

5. Chia Seed Pudding with Berries:
In a bowl or jar, combine chia seeds with
unsweetened almond or coconut milk.
Add a little vanilla extract and a natural sweetener,
such as stevia or monk fruit sweetener, and stir.

Put the mixture in the fridge for several hours or
even overnight to thicken.
Add some fresh berries on top for antioxidants and
extra sweetness.

6. Almond Butter and Banana Slices:
Spread almond butter on banana slices for a quick
and satisfying sweet treat.
Almond butter provides healthy fats and protein,
while bananas offer natural sweetness and
potassium.

7. Dark Chocolate Covered Almonds:
Dip raw almonds in melted dark chocolate and
allow to harden on a baking sheet lined with
parchment paper.

Dark chocolate contains antioxidants and may have beneficial effects on insulin sensitivity, while almonds provide protein and healthy fats.

8. Homemade Trail Mix:

Combine a variety of nuts, seeds, and unsweetened dried fruits like raisins, apricots, and cranberries. Portion into small containers for a convenient and satisfying snack.
Nuts and seeds provide protein and healthy fats, while dried fruits add natural sweetness and fiber.

9. Coconut Date Energy Balls:

Blend pitted dates with shredded coconut, almond flour, and a splash of vanilla extract in a food processor until a sticky dough forms.
Roll mixture into bite-sized balls and coat with additional shredded coconut if desired.
Dates provide natural sweetness and fiber, while coconut adds flavor and texture.

10. **Cinnamon Roasted Almonds:**
Add a dash of cinnamon and a drizzle of honey or
maple syrup to raw almonds.
Roast until fragrant and golden in the oven.
Let cool completely before serving.
Rich in fiber, healthy fats, and protein, almonds
make a filling and wholesome snack choice.

Tips for Sweet Treats on a PCOS Diet:

Choose Whole Foods: Option for desserts made
with whole, minimally processed ingredients to
maximize nutrient intake and minimize added
sugars and unhealthy fats.

Use Natural Sweeteners Sparingly: Incorporate
natural sweeteners like honey, maple syrup, stevia,
or dates in moderation to sweeten treats without
causing blood sugar spikes.

Focus on Fiber and Protein: Include sources of
fiber and protein in sweet treats to slow down the
absorption of sugar into the bloodstream and
promote satiety.

Portion Control: Be mindful of portion sizes to avoid overindulging, especially with calorie-dense treats like nuts, seeds, and dried fruits.

Experiment with Flavors: Get creative with flavor combinations and ingredients to satisfy cravings without compromising on health.

Indulgent desserts made with PCOS-friendly ingredients

PCOS (polycystic ovarian syndrome) patients must pay close attention to their diet, particularly when it comes to dessert consumption. But eating sweets doesn't have to be forbidden. You can satiate your sweet tooth and support your health objectives by using PCOS-friendly ingredients in your dessert recipes. The following decadent dessert ideas are suitable for a PCOS diet:

Almond Flour Brownies: Swap traditional flour with almond flour to reduce the glycemic index and increase protein and healthy fats. Use a natural sweetener like stevia or monk fruit instead of refined sugar.

Avocado Chocolate Mousse: Avocado provides healthy fats and creamy texture while cocoa powder adds rich chocolate flavor. Sweeten with a small amount of honey or maple syrup for a deliciously guilt-free treat.

Coconut Flour Pancakes with Berries: Coconut flour is low in carbs and high in fiber, making it an excellent choice for PCOS-friendly desserts. Top fluffy coconut flour pancakes with fresh berries and a drizzle of sugar-free syrup for a delightful breakfast or dessert option.

Greek Yogurt Parfait: Layer Greek yogurt with chopped nuts, seeds, and a sprinkle of cinnamon for a satisfying dessert packed with protein and probiotics. Add a few berries or a teaspoon of unsweetened cocoa powder for extra flavor.

Chia Seed Pudding: Mix chia seeds with unsweetened almond milk and vanilla extract, then let it sit overnight to thicken into a pudding-like consistency. Stir in your favorite low-glycemic fruits like berries or sliced peaches for a nutritious and indulgent dessert.

Baked Apples with Cinnamon: Core apples and fill them with a mixture of chopped nuts, cinnamon, and a drizzle of honey or maple syrup. Bake until tender for a warm and comforting dessert that's naturally sweet and satisfying.

Pumpkin Spice Energy Balls: Combine pumpkin puree, almond flour, nut butter, and warm spices like cinnamon and nutmeg. Roll into bite-sized balls and chill until firm for a convenient and flavorful snack or dessert option.

Coconut Milk Ice Cream: Make your own dairy-free ice cream using coconut milk as the base. Sweeten with stevia or monk fruit and add flavorings like vanilla extract, cocoa powder, or fresh fruit for a refreshing and indulgent treat.

Protein-Packed Banana Bread: Use a combination of almond flour and protein powder to create a moist and flavorful banana bread that's perfect for satisfying cravings without spiking blood sugar levels. Enjoy as a snack or dessert with a dollop of Greek yogurt on top.

Dark Chocolate Bark with Nuts and Seeds: Melt dark chocolate and spread it onto a baking sheet. Sprinkle with chopped nuts, seeds, and a pinch of sea salt before chilling until set. Break into pieces for a decadent and nutrient-rich dessert option.

CHAPTER EIGHT

Beverages

Maintaining a healthy diet is crucial for managing Polycystic Ovary Syndrome (PCOS), and choosing the right beverages can play a significant role in supporting hormonal balance and overall well-being. Here are some comprehensive recommendations for beverages that align with a PCOS-friendly diet:

Green Tea: Green tea is rich in antioxidants, particularly catechins, which may help reduce insulin resistance and lower levels of testosterone in women with PCOS. Its low caffeine content makes it a suitable option for those looking to minimize caffeine intake.

Herbal Teas: Herbal teas such as peppermint, spearmint, chamomile, and ginger can offer various health benefits for women with PCOS. Peppermint and spearmint teas may help reduce levels of androgens, while chamomile and ginger teas can aid in digestion and promote relaxation.

Water: Staying hydrated is essential for overall health and hormone regulation. Drinking an adequate amount of water throughout the day can help flush out toxins, support metabolism, and maintain optimal hormone balance. Aim to drink at least 8-10 glasses of water daily.

Coconut Water: Coconut water is a refreshing and hydrating beverage that contains electrolytes such as potassium and magnesium. It can help replenish electrolyte levels and maintain hydration, making it a suitable option for women with PCOS, especially those who engage in physical activity.

Almond Milk: Low in calories and carbs, unsweetened almond milk is a dairy-free substitute for cow's milk. Additionally, it has a lot of calcium and vitamin E, two nutrients that are crucial for PCOS-affected women. Pick varieties without added sugars if you want to avoid them.

Turmeric Latte: Curcumin, an anti-inflammatory and antioxidant compound, is found in turmeric. You can satisfy your taste buds and your health by indulging in a turmeric latte made with unsweetened almond milk, a dash of cinnamon, and a pinch of black pepper to improve absorption.

Vegetable Juices: Freshly squeezed vegetable juices, such as carrot, beet, spinach, and kale juice, can be nutritious additions to a PCOS-friendly diet. These juices are rich in vitamins, minerals, and antioxidants, which can support overall health and hormone balance.

Protein Smoothies: Blend together a combination of protein-rich ingredients such as unsweetened almond milk, Greek yogurt, spinach, avocado, and a scoop of protein powder for a satisfying and nutritious smoothie. Adding low-glycemic fruits like berries or half a banana can provide natural sweetness without causing blood sugar spikes.

Bone Broth: Bone broth is rich in collagen, amino acids, and minerals that support gut health and digestion. Incorporating bone broth into your diet can help reduce inflammation and support hormone balance, making it a beneficial beverage for women with PCOS.

Lemon Water: Starting your day with a glass of warm lemon water can help stimulate digestion,

detoxify the body, and support liver function.
Lemons are also rich in vitamin C, which can help
reduce inflammation and boost immune function.

PCOS-friendly drinks to stay hydrated and energized

For women with Polycystic Ovary Syndrome
(PCOS), maintaining energy and hydration is
crucial for maintaining hormone balance and
general health. Here are a few thorough suggestions
for PCOS-friendly beverages that will keep you
hydrated and alert:

Infused Water: Infusing water with fruits,
vegetables, and herbs can add flavor and nutrients
without added sugars or artificial ingredients. Try
combinations like cucumber and mint, lemon and

ginger, or berries and basil for refreshing and hydrating options.

Coconut Water: Coconut water is naturally rich in electrolytes like potassium, magnesium, and sodium, making it an excellent choice for hydration. It's low in calories and sugar, making it a PCOS-friendly alternative to sugary sports drinks.

Herbal Teas: Herbal teas such as peppermint, spearmint, chamomile, and rooibos are caffeine-free options that can help hydrate and soothe digestion. Peppermint and spearmint teas may also help reduce levels of androgens in women with PCOS.

Green Smoothies: Blend together leafy greens like spinach or kale with low-glycemic fruits like berries, along with a source of protein like Greek yogurt or protein powder. Green smoothies are nutrient-dense and can provide a sustained energy boost without spiking blood sugar levels.

Sparkling Water with Citrus: Adding a splash of citrus juice to sparkling water can create a refreshing and hydrating beverage without added sugars or artificial flavors. Try combinations like sparkling water with lime or grapefruit juice for a zesty twist.

Golden Milk Latte: Golden milk, made with turmeric, ginger, and coconut milk, is a warming and comforting drink that can help reduce inflammation and support hormone balance. Enjoy it warm or cold for a nourishing and energizing beverage option.

Berry Blast Smoothie: Blend together mixed berries like strawberries, blueberries, and raspberries with unsweetened almond milk or coconut water, along with a scoop of protein powder or Greek yogurt for added protein. This vibrant smoothie is packed with antioxidants and can help keep you hydrated and satisfied.

Iced Herbal Tea: Brew herbal teas like hibiscus, chamomile, or lemon balm and chill them in the refrigerator for a refreshing and hydrating iced tea option. Add a squeeze of lemon or a few fresh mint leaves for extra flavor.

Matcha Latte: Matcha is a powdered green tea that is rich in antioxidants and provides a sustained energy boost without the jitters associated with coffee. Enjoy a matcha latte made with unsweetened almond milk or coconut milk for a PCOS-friendly alternative to traditional lattes.

Electrolyte-Rich Smoothie: Blend together coconut water, spinach, banana, and a scoop of protein powder for a hydrating and energizing smoothie that's rich in electrolytes and nutrients. This smoothie is perfect for replenishing electrolytes after exercise or during hot weather.

Smoothie recipes packed with nutrients and flavor

Smoothies are a convenient and delicious way to pack a variety of nutrients into your diet while managing Polycystic Ovary Syndrome (PCOS). Here are some comprehensive smoothie recipes tailored for a PCOS-friendly diet, packed with nutrients and flavor:

Berry Blast Smoothie:

Ingredients: 1 cup mixed berries (strawberries, blueberries, raspberries), 1/2 banana, 1 cup spinach, 1/2 cup unsweetened almond milk, 1 tablespoon chia seeds, 1 scoop protein powder (optional).
Instructions: Blend all ingredients until smooth. Add more almond milk if needed for desired consistency. Serve and enjoy!

Green Goddess Smoothie:

Ingredients: 1 cup coconut water, ice cubes, 1/2 avocado, 1/2 cucumber, 1/2 green apple, 1 tablespoon fresh ginger, and 1 tablespoon lemon juice.
Guidelines: Mix every ingredient until it's smooth. If you want a colder consistency, add ice cubes. Transfer into a glass and decorate with a cucumber or lemon slice.

Creamy Coconut Pineapple Smoothie:

Ingredients: 1/2 cup frozen pineapple chunks, 1/2 cup Greek yogurt, 1/2 cup coconut milk, 1 tablespoon unsweetened shredded coconut, ice cubes, and optional 1 tablespoon honey or maple syrup.

Instructions: Blend until creamy and smooth, combining all ingredients. If you would like a thicker texture, add ice cubes. Transfer into a glass and garnish with extra shredded coconut.

Tropical Turmeric Smoothie:

Ingredients: 1 cup frozen mango chunks, 1/2 banana, 1/2 tsp ground cinnamon, 1/2 tsp turmeric powder, 1 tablespoon chia seeds, and 1 cup unsweetened almond milk or coconut water.

Directions: Process until smooth, blending all ingredients. If necessary, add extra almond milk or coconut water to adjust the sweetness and consistency. Garnish with a little cinnamon before serving.

Chocolate Almond Butter Protein Smoothie:

Ingredients: 1/2 banana, 1 cup unsweetened almond milk, 1 scoop chocolate protein powder, 1 tablespoon unsweetened cocoa powder, and ice cubes.

Guidelines: Blend each ingredient until it becomes creamy and smooth. If you would like a thicker texture, add ice cubes. Pour into a glass and savor this decadent but healthful dessert.

Banana-Berry Oatmeal Smoothie:

Ingredients: 1/2 cup of mixed berries (strawberries, blueberries, and raspberries), 1/2 banana, 1/4 cup of rolled oats, 1/2 cup of Greek yogurt, 1/2 cup of unsweetened almond milk, and 1 tablespoon of optional honey or maple syrup.

Directions: Process until smooth, blending all ingredients. If desired, adjust sweetness by adding extra honey or maple syrup. For extra texture, top with a sprinkle of oats and serve.

Peanut Butter Banana Protein Smoothie:

Ingredients: 1/2 banana, 1/2 cup unsweetened almond milk, 1/2 tablespoon natural peanut butter, 1/2 scoop protein powder with vanilla, 1/2 tablespoon flax seeds, and ice cubes.
Guidelines: Blend each ingredient until it becomes creamy and smooth. If you would like a thicker texture, add ice cubes. Transfer into a glass and decorate with a flaxseed or a slice of banana.

Detoxifying Green Smoothie:

Ingredients: 1/2 cup cucumber, 1/2 cup green apple, 1/2 juiced lemon, 1 tablespoon fresh parsley, 1 tablespoon chia seeds, 1/2 cup water or coconut water, and ice cubes.
Directions: Process until smooth, blending all ingredients. If you want a colder consistency, add ice cubes. Pour into a glass, then savor this cooling, cleansing smoothie.

These tasty, nutrient-dense smoothie recipes allow you to support your health goals while having delicious, fulfilling drinks. Add them to your PCOS diet. Try out various ingredient combinations to discover which flavors and textures you prefer. For the best possible health effects, always choose premium, whole food ingredients and stay away from adding a lot of sugar or artificial additives.

Herbal teas and infusions for hormonal balance

Herbal teas and infusions offer natural remedies that can help support hormonal balance, which is essential for managing Polycystic Ovary Syndrome (PCOS). Here are some comprehensive herbal teas and infusions tailored for a PCOS-friendly diet:

Spearmint Tea: Spearmint tea has been studied for its potential to reduce levels of androgens, such as testosterone, in women with PCOS. Drinking spearmint tea regularly may help alleviate symptoms like hirsutism (excess hair growth) and acne associated with elevated androgen levels.

Peppermint Tea: Peppermint tea not only has a refreshing flavor but also contains anti-androgenic properties that can help regulate hormone levels in women with PCOS. Enjoying a cup of peppermint tea after meals may aid digestion and promote hormonal balance.

Chamomile Tea: Chamomile tea is known for its calming effects on the body and mind. It can help reduce stress and anxiety, which are common concerns for women with PCOS. Drinking chamomile tea before bedtime may improve sleep quality and support overall hormone regulation.

Raspberry Leaf Tea: Raspberry leaf tea is rich in nutrients like vitamins C and B, as well as minerals like magnesium and potassium. It is believed to support reproductive health and hormonal balance by toning the uterus and regulating menstrual cycles. Raspberry leaf tea is often recommended for women with PCOS who experience irregular periods.

Nettle Leaf Tea: Nettle leaf tea is a nourishing herbal infusion that is high in vitamins, minerals, and antioxidants. It is particularly beneficial for women with PCOS due to its ability to support liver function and detoxification, which can help regulate hormone levels and improve overall health.

Ginger Tea: Ginger tea is renowned for its anti-inflammatory and digestive properties. It can help reduce inflammation in the body, which is often elevated in women with PCOS. Drinking ginger tea regularly may also support healthy metabolism and digestion, promoting hormonal balance.

Licorice Root Tea: Licorice root tea has adaptogenic properties, meaning it helps the body adapt to stress and maintain balance. It can support adrenal function and cortisol regulation, which are important for managing stress and hormone levels in women with PCOS. However, it should be consumed in moderation due to its potential to raise blood pressure.

Cinnamon Infusion: Cinnamon is a warming spice that may help improve insulin sensitivity and regulate blood sugar levels in women with PCOS. Steep a cinnamon stick in hot water to create a flavorful infusion that can be enjoyed throughout the day.

Dandelion Root Tea: Dandelion root tea is a gentle diuretic that can help support liver health and detoxification. It may aid in hormonal balance by promoting the elimination of excess hormones and toxins from the body, making it a beneficial beverage for women with PCOS.

Fennel Seed Infusion: Fennel seeds contain compounds that mimic estrogen in the body, making them potentially useful for women with PCOS who have hormonal imbalances. Steep fennel seeds in hot water to create a soothing infusion that can be enjoyed after meals or as a bedtime beverage.

By adding these herbal teas and infusions to your diet, you can manage the hormonal balance of your PCOS, lessen symptoms, and enhance your general health. When starting new herbal remedies, always choose organic, high-quality herbs and get medical advice, especially if you have any underlying health conditions or are on medication.

CHAPTER NINE

Special Dietary Considerations

Particular dietary considerations are needed for PCOS in order to support overall health and help manage symptoms. The following are extensive dietary recommendations designed for a PCOS-friendly diet:

Focus on Low-Glycemic Foods: Choose carbohydrates that have a low glycemic index to help stabilize blood sugar levels and reduce insulin resistance, a common issue in women with PCOS. Opt for whole grains like quinoa, brown rice, and oats, as well as legumes, fruits, and vegetables.

Balanced Macronutrient Intake: Aim to include a balance of protein, carbohydrates, and healthy fats in each meal to support satiety and blood sugar control. Include lean proteins such as chicken, fish, tofu, and legumes, along with healthy fats like avocados, nuts, seeds, and olive oil.

Limit Added Sugars and Refined Carbohydrates: Minimize intake of foods and beverages that are high in added sugars and refined carbohydrates, as they can contribute to insulin resistance and hormone imbalances. Avoid sugary snacks, sodas, baked goods, and processed foods whenever possible.

Increase Fiber Intake: Fiber-rich foods can help improve digestion, promote fullness, and regulate blood sugar levels. Include plenty of fruits, vegetables, whole grains, legumes, nuts, and seeds in your diet to meet your fiber needs and support digestive health.

Choose Healthy Sources of Fats: Option for unsaturated fats found in foods like avocados, nuts, seeds, olive oil, and fatty fish like salmon and mackerel. These fats can help reduce inflammation and support hormone production and balance.

Moderate Intake of Dairy Products: Some women with PCOS may be sensitive to dairy products, which can exacerbate symptoms like acne and inflammation. Consider reducing or eliminating dairy from your diet and choose dairy alternatives like almond milk, coconut yogurt, or cashew cheese instead.

Include Anti-Inflammatory Foods: Incorporate foods rich in anti-inflammatory nutrients, such as omega-3 fatty acids, antioxidants, and phytonutrients, to help reduce inflammation and support overall health. Include fatty fish, leafy greens, berries, turmeric, ginger, and garlic in your diet regularly.

Stay Hydrated: Drink plenty of water throughout the day to stay hydrated and support metabolism, digestion, and hormone balance. Herbal teas, infused water, and coconut water are also excellent options for staying hydrated without added sugars or caffeine.

Practice Portion Control: Pay attention to portion sizes and avoid overeating, as excess weight can exacerbate symptoms of PCOS. Focus on eating until you feel satisfied rather than overly full, and listen to your body's hunger and fullness cues.

Consider Supplements: Talk to your healthcare provider about potentially beneficial supplements for PCOS, such as omega-3 fatty acids, magnesium, vitamin D, and inositol. These supplements may help support hormone balance, insulin sensitivity, and overall health.

By following these special dietary considerations, you can help manage symptoms, support hormone balance, and improve overall well-being while living with PCOS. Remember that individual dietary needs may vary, so it's essential to work with a healthcare provider or registered dietitian to create a personalized nutrition plan that meets your specific needs and goals.

Gluten-free and dairy-free options for those with sensitivities

Managing Polycystic Ovary Syndrome (PCOS) often involves dietary adjustments, particularly for individuals with sensitivities to gluten and dairy. Here are some comprehensive gluten-free and dairy-free options tailored for a PCOS-friendly diet:

Quinoa Salad: Quinoa is a gluten-free whole grain that is rich in protein and fiber, making it an excellent base for salads. Combine cooked quinoa with chopped vegetables like cucumber, tomato, bell peppers, and avocado. Dress with olive oil, lemon juice, and herbs for a flavorful and nutritious meal.

Zucchini Noodles with Pesto: Spiralized zucchini makes a delicious gluten-free alternative to pasta. Toss zucchini noodles with dairy-free pesto made from basil, pine nuts, garlic, nutritional yeast, and olive oil. Top with cherry tomatoes and grilled chicken or tofu for added protein.

Coconut Curry with Vegetables: Coconut milk is a creamy and dairy-free alternative to traditional cream in curries. Make a flavorful coconut curry with mixed vegetables like bell peppers, carrots, and broccoli. Add protein sources such as chickpeas, tofu, or shrimp, and serve over brown rice or quinoa.

Gluten-Free Oatmeal with Almond Milk: Start your day with a hearty bowl of gluten-free oatmeal made with unsweetened almond milk. Top with fresh berries, sliced banana, and a sprinkle of nuts or seeds for added flavor and nutrition. Avoid pre-packaged oatmeal blends that may contain gluten.

Stir-Fried Tofu with Vegetables: Stir-fry tofu with an assortment of colorful vegetables like bell peppers, snap peas, and mushrooms. Season with gluten-free tamari sauce, garlic, and ginger for a flavorful and satisfying meal. Serve over brown rice or cauliflower rice for a low-carb option.

Dairy-Free Smoothie Bowl: Blend together frozen mixed berries, spinach, banana, and unsweetened almond milk to create a thick and creamy smoothie base. Pour into a bowl and top with gluten-free granola, sliced fruit, coconut flakes, and chia seeds for a nutritious and satisfying breakfast or snack.

Gluten-Free Cauliflower Pizza: Use a gluten-free cauliflower pizza crust as a base for your favorite pizza toppings. Top with dairy-free tomato sauce, vegetables, and dairy-free cheese alternatives like almond or cashew cheese. Bake until crispy and golden for a delicious and satisfying meal.

Salmon with Roasted Vegetables: Roast a filet of salmon seasoned with herbs and spices alongside a medley of roasted vegetables such as Brussels sprouts, sweet potatoes, and cauliflower. Drizzle with olive oil and balsamic vinegar for a flavorful and nutrient-rich dinner option.

Chia Seed Pudding: Make a dairy-free chia seed pudding by combining chia seeds with unsweetened almond milk, vanilla extract, and a natural sweetener like maple syrup or stevia. Let it sit in the refrigerator overnight to thicken, then top with fresh fruit, nuts, and seeds before serving.

Gluten-Free Banana Bread: Bake a gluten-free banana bread using a blend of gluten-free flours such as almond flour, coconut flour, and tapioca flour. Replace dairy ingredients with dairy-free alternatives like coconut oil and almond milk. Enjoy a slice as a satisfying snack or dessert option.

These gluten-free and dairy-free options provide delicious and nutritious choices for individuals with sensitivities while following a PCOS-friendly diet. Experiment with different ingredients and recipes to find combinations that suit your taste preferences and dietary needs.

Vegetarian and vegan recipes suitable for PCOS diets

Following a vegetarian or vegan diet can offer numerous health benefits for individuals managing Polycystic Ovary Syndrome (PCOS). Here are some vegetarian and vegan recipes tailored for a PCOS-friendly diet:

Vegetable Stir-Fry with Tofu: Stir-frying a colorful array of vegetables like bell peppers, broccoli, carrots, and snap peas with tofu provides a nutritious and protein-rich meal. Season with garlic, ginger, and gluten-free tamari sauce for flavor. For extra fiber, serve over quinoa or brown rice.

Chickpea Salad: Add diced cucumber, tomato, red onion, and parsley to cooked chickpeas. Toss with lemon juice, olive oil, salt, and pepper for a light and high-protein salad. Serve over mixed greens or use whole-grain tortillas as a satisfying wrap.

Vegan Lentil Soup: Make a hearty lentil soup by simmering lentils with carrots, celery, onion, garlic, and vegetable broth. Season with cumin, coriander, and smoked paprika for depth of flavor. Serve with a side of gluten-free bread or crackers for a satisfying meal.

Quinoa and Black Bean Burrito Bowl: Create a burrito bowl by layering cooked quinoa with seasoned black beans, roasted sweet potatoes, sautéed bell peppers and onions, avocado slices, and salsa. Garnish with fresh cilantro and a squeeze of lime for a zesty and nutritious meal.

Stuffed Bell Peppers with Quinoa and Spinach: Stuff halved bell peppers with a mixture of cooked quinoa, sautéed spinach, diced tomatoes, black beans, corn, and spices. Bake until tender for a flavorful and protein-rich dish. Top with dairy-free cheese alternative if desired.

Vegan Chickpea Curry: Prepare a fragrant chickpea curry by simmering chickpeas with coconut milk, diced tomatoes, onion, garlic, ginger, and curry spices. Add in vegetables like cauliflower, peas, and spinach for extra nutrition. For a filling supper, serve over quinoa or brown rice.

Vegetable and Tofu Stir-Fried Noodles: Stir-fry tofu with a colorful mix of vegetables such as bell peppers, broccoli, carrots, and snow peas. Toss with cooked rice noodles and a flavorful sauce made from tamari, sesame oil, garlic, and chili paste. Garnish with chopped peanuts and cilantro for added texture and flavor.

Vegan Buddha Bowl: Create a nourishing Buddha bowl by combining cooked grains like quinoa or brown rice with roasted vegetables, marinated tofu or tempeh, avocado slices, and a drizzle of tahini dressing. Customize with your favorite vegetables and toppings for a balanced and satisfying meal.

Vegan Spinach and Mushroom Omelette: Make a vegan omelet using chickpea flour as the base, and fill it with sautéed spinach, mushrooms, onions, and dairy-free cheese alternative. Serve with a side of roasted potatoes or a mixed greens salad for a hearty breakfast or brunch option.

Vegan Chocolate Avocado Mousse: Indulge in a creamy and decadent dessert by blending ripe avocados with cocoa powder, maple syrup, vanilla extract, and a pinch of salt until smooth and creamy. Chill in the refrigerator until set, then serve topped with fresh berries and chopped nuts for added texture.

These vegetarian and vegan recipes offer flavorful and nutritious options for individuals following a PCOS-friendly diet. Experiment with different ingredients and flavors to create delicious meals that support your health and well-being.

Low-carb adaptations for managing insulin resistance

Managing insulin resistance is a key aspect of a PCOS diet, and adopting a low-carb approach can be beneficial for improving insulin sensitivity and managing symptoms. Here are some low-carb adaptations tailored specifically for individuals with PCOS:

Replace Grains with Non-Starchy Vegetables:
Swap out grains like rice, pasta, and bread with
non-starchy vegetables such as spinach, broccoli,
cauliflower, zucchini, and bell peppers. These
vegetables are low in carbs and high in fiber,
helping to stabilize blood sugar levels and improve
insulin sensitivity.

Choose Low-Glycemic Fruits: Option for
low-glycemic fruits such as berries (strawberries,
blueberries, raspberries), cherries, apples, and pears,
which have a lower impact on blood sugar levels

compared to high-glycemic fruits like bananas,
grapes, and melons. Enjoy them in moderation as
part of a balanced meal or snack.

Include Lean Proteins: Incorporate lean sources of
protein into your meals to help stabilize blood sugar
levels and promote satiety. Choose options like
skinless poultry, fish, tofu, tempeh, eggs, and

legumes. Protein-rich foods can help balance out the effects of carbohydrates and prevent spikes in insulin.

Healthy Fats as a Fuel Source: Emphasize healthy fats as a primary fuel source to provide sustained energy and promote satiety. Include foods like avocados, nuts, seeds, olives, coconut oil, and fatty fish in your diet. Healthy fats are low in carbs and can help stabilize blood sugar levels by slowing down the absorption of glucose.

Mindful Snacking: Choose low-carb snacks that are high in protein and healthy fats to help keep blood sugar levels stable between meals. Snack options may include nuts, seeds, Greek yogurt (if tolerated), cheese sticks, hard-boiled eggs, and vegetable sticks with hummus or guacamole.

Limit Added Sugars and Processed Foods:
Minimize intake of added sugars, refined
carbohydrates, and processed foods, as they can
contribute to insulin resistance and exacerbate
symptoms of PCOS. Avoid sugary snacks, sodas,
candies, baked goods, and processed snacks
whenever possible.

Portion Control: Observe portion sizes and refrain
from overindulging, even when consuming
low-carb foods. Even when consumed in excess,
calories from low-carb sources can exacerbate
insulin resistance and cause weight gain. Pay
attention to your body's signals of hunger and
fullness and practice portion control.

Stay Hydrated: Drink plenty of water throughout
the day to help flush out toxins and support
metabolism. Hydration is essential for maintaining
overall health and can also aid in regulating blood
sugar levels and insulin sensitivity.

Regular Physical Activity: Include exercise on a
regular basis in your regimen to help control your

weight and enhance insulin sensitivity. To promote general health and wellbeing, try to incorporate cardiovascular, strength, and flexibility exercises into your routine.

Monitor Blood Sugar Levels: Consider monitoring your blood sugar levels regularly, especially if you have insulin resistance or diabetes. Keeping track of your blood sugar levels can help you understand how different foods and lifestyle choices affect your body and allow you to make informed decisions about your diet and health.

CHAPTER TEN

Lifestyle Tips for Managing PCOS

Polycystic Ovary Syndrome (PCOS) is a complex condition that can affect various aspects of a woman's health. Alongside medical treatment, adopting healthy lifestyle habits can play a crucial role in managing PCOS symptoms and improving overall well-being. Here are some comprehensive lifestyle tips for managing PCOS:

Regular Exercise: Engage in regular physical activity to help improve insulin sensitivity, manage weight, and reduce the risk of complications associated with PCOS, such as type 2 diabetes and heart disease. Aim for at least 150 minutes of moderate-intensity exercise or 75 minutes of vigorous-intensity exercise per week, along with strength training exercises two or more days a week.

Healthy Diet: Follow a balanced and nutritious diet that focuses on whole, unprocessed foods such as fruits, vegetables, lean proteins, whole grains, and healthy fats. Opt for low-glycemic index foods to help stabilize blood sugar levels and reduce insulin resistance. Limit consumption of sugary foods, refined carbohydrates, and processed foods, which can exacerbate PCOS symptoms.

Manage Stress: Chronic stress can worsen PCOS symptoms by increasing cortisol levels and disrupting hormone balance. Incorporate stress-reducing techniques into your daily routine, such as mindfulness meditation, deep breathing exercises, yoga, tai chi, or spending time in nature. Make self-care activities that enhance wellbeing and relaxation a priority.

Adequate Sleep: Prioritize getting enough quality sleep each night, as inadequate sleep can negatively impact hormone regulation and exacerbate PCOS symptoms. Aim for 7-9 hours of uninterrupted sleep per night and establish a consistent sleep schedule by going to bed and waking up at the same time each day.

Maintain a Healthy Weight: Achieving and maintaining a healthy weight can help improve hormone balance and reduce the severity of PCOS symptoms. Focus on gradual, sustainable weight loss through a combination of healthy eating, regular exercise, and lifestyle modifications. Consult with a healthcare provider or registered dietitian for personalized weight management guidance.

Regular Medical Check-ups: Schedule regular medical check-ups with your healthcare provider to monitor your PCOS symptoms and overall health. Discuss any concerns or changes in symptoms during these appointments and work together to develop an individualized treatment plan that addresses your specific needs and goals.

Keep Yourself Informed: Gain the knowledge necessary to make wise decisions regarding your health by becoming knowledgeable about PCOS and its management techniques. Keep abreast on the most recent findings, available therapies, and suggested lifestyle changes for managing PCOS. Join online forums or support groups to meet other PCOS sufferers and exchange stories and guidance.

Limit Exposure to Environmental Toxins: Minimize exposure to environmental toxins and endocrine-disrupting chemicals found in everyday products such as plastics, cosmetics, cleaning supplies, and pesticides. Choose natural and organic products whenever possible and opt for environmentally friendly alternatives to reduce your exposure to harmful chemicals.

Supportive Relationships: Surround yourself with supportive friends, family members, and healthcare providers who understand and respect your journey with PCOS. Seek out support groups or counseling services if needed to connect with others who can offer encouragement, understanding, and advice.

Be Patient and Persistent: Managing PCOS is a journey that requires patience, persistence, and dedication. Understand that progress may take time, and setbacks are a natural part of the process. Stay committed to your health goals and celebrate your achievements, no matter how small they may seem.

Importance of regular exercise for PCOS management

Frequent exercise is essential for managing Polycystic Ovary Syndrome (PCOS) because it can help with overall health improvement, symptom relief, and lowering the chance of PCOS complications. Here are a few thorough justifications for why consistent exercise is crucial for managing PCOS:

Improves Insulin Sensitivity: Insulin resistance is a common characteristic of PCOS, leading to elevated insulin levels in the blood. Regular exercise helps improve insulin sensitivity, allowing the body to use insulin more effectively to regulate blood sugar levels. This can help lower insulin levels, reduce the risk of type 2 diabetes, and improve metabolic health in women with PCOS.

Aids in Weight Management: Many women with PCOS struggle with weight management due to hormonal imbalances and metabolic issues. Regular exercise, especially a combination of cardiovascular exercise and strength training, can help promote weight loss or weight maintenance by increasing calorie expenditure, building lean muscle mass, and boosting metabolism. Even modest weight loss can lead to significant improvements in PCOS symptoms and overall health.

Reduces Androgen Levels: Elevated levels of androgens, such as testosterone, are often associated with PCOS and can contribute to symptoms like hirsutism (excess hair growth) and acne. Exercise has been shown to help reduce circulating androgen levels in women with PCOS, potentially improving symptoms and promoting hormonal balance.

Promotes Hormonal Balance: Regular exercise can help regulate hormone levels in women with PCOS by promoting the production of endorphins, serotonin, and other neurotransmitters that help regulate mood and stress. This can help alleviate symptoms of depression, anxiety, and mood swings commonly experienced by women with PCOS.

Supports Menstrual Regularity: Irregular menstrual cycles are a hallmark feature of PCOS, often due to hormonal imbalances and ovulatory dysfunction. Exercise can help regulate menstrual cycles by promoting hormonal balance and improving ovulation. Women with PCOS who engage in regular exercise may experience more regular menstrual cycles and improved fertility.

Reduces Cardiovascular Risk: Women with PCOS are at an increased risk of cardiovascular disease due to factors such as insulin resistance, obesity, and dyslipidemia (abnormal lipid levels). Regular exercise can help reduce cardiovascular risk factors by improving insulin sensitivity, lowering blood pressure, reducing cholesterol levels, and promoting heart health.

Enhances Mood and Well-Being: Exercise has been shown to have numerous psychological benefits, including reducing stress, anxiety, and depression, and improving mood and overall well-being. Women with PCOS may experience improved mental health and quality of life by incorporating regular exercise into their routine.

Supports Bone Health: Women with PCOS are at a higher risk of osteoporosis due to hormonal imbalances and low estrogen levels. Weight-bearing exercises such as walking, jogging, dancing, and strength training can help improve bone density and reduce the risk of osteoporosis and fractures.

Improves Energy Levels and Fatigue: Many women with PCOS experience fatigue and low energy levels, which can impact daily functioning and quality of life. Regular exercise can help boost energy levels, reduce fatigue, and improve overall vitality by increasing circulation, oxygen delivery, and mitochondrial function.

Empowers Self-Management: Incorporating regular exercise into a PCOS management plan empowers women to take an active role in their health and well-being. By adopting a consistent exercise routine, women with PCOS can gain a sense of control over their symptoms, improve self-esteem, and enhance their overall quality of life.

In summary, exercise on a regular basis is essential for managing PCOS because it has so many positive effects on the body, hormones, mind, and emotions. It is advised that women with PCOS take part in a range of enjoyable, long-term physical activities. A healthcare provider or certified fitness professional should be consulted in order to create a personalized exercise program that fits your needs, preferences, and goals while taking into account any underlying medical conditions or limitations.

Stress-reduction techniques and their impact on hormonal balance

Stress reduction techniques play a vital role in managing Polycystic Ovary Syndrome (PCOS) by helping to alleviate symptoms, improve hormonal balance, and enhance overall well-being. Here are some comprehensive stress-reduction techniques and their impact on hormonal balance for individuals following a PCOS diet:

Mindfulness Meditation: Mindfulness meditation involves focusing on the present moment without judgment, allowing individuals to become more aware of their thoughts, feelings, and bodily sensations. Regular practice of mindfulness meditation has been shown to reduce stress levels, lower cortisol (stress hormone) levels, and improve hormonal balance in women with PCOS.

Deep Breathing Exercises: Deep breathing exercises, such as diaphragmatic breathing or belly breathing, help activate the body's relaxation response and promote a sense of calmness and relaxation. Deep breathing can reduce sympathetic nervous system activity, lower cortisol levels, and improve hormonal balance by modulating the stress response.

Yoga: Yoga combines physical postures, breathing exercises, and meditation techniques to promote relaxation, flexibility, and mindfulness. Practicing yoga regularly has been associated with reduced stress, anxiety, and depression, as well as improvements in hormonal balance, menstrual regularity, and fertility in women with PCOS.

Tai Chi: Tai Chi is a gentle form of mind-body exercise that involves slow, flowing movements and deep breathing. Studies have shown that practicing Tai Chi can reduce stress, improve mood, and enhance hormonal balance by regulating the hypothalamic-pituitary-adrenal (HPA) axis and reducing cortisol levels in individuals with PCOS.

Progressive Muscle Relaxation: Progressive muscle relaxation involves systematically tensing and relaxing different muscle groups in the body to induce a state of deep relaxation. This technique can help reduce muscle tension, alleviate stress, and promote hormonal balance by lowering cortisol levels and activating the parasympathetic nervous system.

Guided Imagery: Guided imagery involves using mental imagery to evoke feelings of relaxation, calmness, and well-being. Visualization techniques can help reduce stress, anxiety, and depression, as well as improve hormonal balance by promoting positive emotions and reducing cortisol levels in women with PCOS.

Biofeedback: Biofeedback is a technique that helps individuals learn to control physiological responses such as heart rate, blood pressure, and muscle tension through mental focus and relaxation techniques. Biofeedback training can help reduce stress levels, improve mood, and enhance hormonal balance by promoting self-regulation of the autonomic nervous system.

Aromatherapy: Aromatherapy involves using essential oils extracted from plants to promote relaxation, reduce stress, and improve mood. Certain essential oils, such as lavender, chamomile, and bergamot, have been shown to have calming effects and can help alleviate symptoms of stress and anxiety, promoting hormonal balance in women with PCOS.

Journaling: Journaling involves writing down thoughts, feelings, and experiences as a form of self-expression and reflection. Keeping a journal can help individuals process emotions, identify stress triggers, and develop coping strategies to manage stress more effectively, leading to improved hormonal balance and overall well-being.

Spending Time in Nature: Spending time in nature, also known as ecotherapy or nature therapy, has been shown to reduce stress, improve mood, and enhance overall well-being. Activities such as walking in the park, hiking in the mountains, or gardening can help lower cortisol levels, promote relaxation, and restore hormonal balance in women with PCOS.

Sleep hygiene practices for optimizing PCOS symptoms

Sleep hygiene practices play a crucial role in optimizing symptoms and managing Polycystic Ovary Syndrome (PCOS). Quality sleep is essential for hormone regulation, metabolism, and overall well-being. Here are some comprehensive sleep hygiene practices tailored for individuals following a PCOS diet:

Create a Regular Sleep Schedule: Even on weekends, create a consistent sleep schedule by going to bed and waking up at the same time every day. Maintaining consistency improves the quality of sleep and helps the body's internal clock.

Establish a Calm Bedtime Routine: Set up a calming routine for before bed to let your body know when it's time to wind down and get ready for sleep. Stress can be reduced and relaxation can be encouraged by engaging in activities like reading, having a warm bath, doing relaxation techniques, or listening to relaxing music.

Limit Screen Time Before Bed: Limit the amount of time you spend using electronics before bed, including computers, televisions, tablets, and smartphones. Screen blue light can interfere with melatonin production and cause sleep patterns to be disturbed. Try to switch off electronics an hour or more before going to bed.

Establish a Comfortable Sleep Environment: Keep your bedroom quiet, dark, and cold to promote restful sleep. To filter out light, use blackout curtains or an eye mask; to block out unwanted noise, use white noise machines or earplugs. Invest in pillows that offer sufficient support and a comfy mattress.

Limit Caffeine and Stimulants: Avoid consuming caffeine and stimulants such as coffee, tea, soda, and energy drinks in the late afternoon and evening. These substances can interfere with sleep quality and disrupt the sleep-wake cycle, making it harder to fall asleep and stay asleep.

Avoid Heavy Meals and Alcohol Before Bed:
Refrain from consuming heavy meals, spicy foods, and alcoholic beverages close to bedtime, as they can cause discomfort, indigestion, and disrupt sleep. Instead, opt for a light snack if you're hungry, and avoid large meals within two to three hours of bedtime.

Exercise Regularly: Engage in regular physical activity during the day, as exercise can help improve sleep quality and promote relaxation. Aim for at least 30 minutes of moderate-intensity exercise most days of the week, but avoid vigorous exercise too close to bedtime, as it may interfere with sleep.

Manage Stress and Anxiety: Practice stress-reduction techniques such as deep breathing exercises, mindfulness meditation, or progressive muscle relaxation to help calm the mind and body before bedtime. Managing stress and anxiety can help promote better sleep quality and improve overall well-being.

Limit Naps During the Day: While short naps can be beneficial for some individuals, excessive daytime napping can disrupt nighttime sleep patterns. If you need to nap during the day, aim for a short nap of 20-30 minutes and avoid napping too close to bedtime.

Seek Professional Help if Needed: If you continue to experience difficulty sleeping despite practicing good sleep hygiene, consider seeking help from a healthcare provider or sleep specialist. They can evaluate your sleep patterns, identify any underlying sleep disorders or medical conditions, and recommend appropriate treatment options.

Glossary of terms related to PCOS and nutrition

Polycystic Ovary Syndrome (PCOS): A hormonal disorder common among women of reproductive age, characterized by irregular menstrual cycles, ovarian cysts, and symptoms such as hirsutism (excess hair growth), acne, and weight gain.

Insulin Resistance: A condition in which cells become less responsive to the effects of insulin, leading to elevated insulin levels in the blood. Insulin resistance is a common feature of PCOS and can contribute to weight gain, metabolic dysfunction, and hormonal imbalances.

The Glycemic Index (GI) quantifies the rate at which a food high in carbohydrates raises blood sugar levels. High-GI foods cause a sudden spike in blood sugar levels, whereas low-GI foods are absorbed and digested more slowly, increasing blood sugar levels gradually.

Macronutrients: Nutrients that provide calories and are required in large amounts in the diet, including carbohydrates, proteins, and fats. Balancing macronutrient intake is essential for managing PCOS and supporting overall health.

Micronutrients: Essential vitamins and minerals that are required in smaller amounts in the diet but are essential for various physiological functions. Micronutrients play a crucial role in hormone regulation, metabolism, and overall well-being.

Androgens: Male sex hormones produced in small amounts by the ovaries and adrenal glands in women. Elevated levels of androgens are a common characteristic of PCOS and can contribute to symptoms such as hirsutism, acne, and irregular menstrual cycles.

Estrogens: Female sex hormones primarily produced by the ovaries that play a key role in reproductive function, bone health, and cardiovascular health. Imbalances in estrogen levels can occur in women with PCOS and may contribute to symptoms such as irregular menstrual cycles and infertility.

Progesterone: A female sex hormone produced by the ovaries that plays a crucial role in regulating the menstrual cycle and supporting pregnancy. Women with PCOS may have irregular menstrual cycles due to disruptions in progesterone production.

Hormone Imbalance: An abnormality in the levels or ratio of hormones in the body, which can disrupt normal physiological functions and contribute to health problems such as PCOS. Hormone imbalances in PCOS often involve elevated levels of androgens, insulin, and luteinizing hormone (LH), and reduced levels of progesterone.

Endocrine Disruptors: Chemical substances found in the environment that can interfere with hormone production, metabolism, and signaling pathways in the body. Exposure to endocrine disruptors may contribute to the development or exacerbation of PCOS symptoms.

Inositol: A group of naturally occurring compounds that play a role in insulin signaling and glucose metabolism. Inositol supplements, particularly myo-inositol and D-chiro-inositol, have been shown to improve insulin sensitivity and menstrual regularity in women with PCOS.

Omega-3 Fatty Acids: Essential fatty acids found in fatty fish, flaxseeds, chia seeds, walnuts, and other sources. Omega-3 fatty acids have anti-inflammatory properties and may help reduce inflammation and improve metabolic health in women with PCOS.

Folate: A B-vitamin that plays a crucial role in DNA synthesis and cell division. Adequate folate intake is important for women with PCOS, especially those who may become pregnant, as it can help reduce the risk of neural tube defects in the developing fetus.

Chromium: A trace mineral that plays a role in insulin signaling and glucose metabolism. Chromium supplements may help improve insulin sensitivity and glucose control in women with PCOS.

Dietary Fiber: Plant-based carbohydrates that are not fully digested or absorbed by the body, providing bulk to the diet and promoting digestive health. High-fiber foods such as fruits, vegetables, whole grains, legumes, and nuts are important components of a PCOS-friendly diet.

This glossary provides an overview of key terms related to PCOS and nutrition, helping individuals better understand the role of diet and lifestyle in managing the condition and promoting overall health and well-being.

CONCLUSION

In conclusion, the "PCOS Diet Cookbook for Beginners" serves as a comprehensive guide for individuals looking to manage their Polycystic Ovary Syndrome (PCOS) through nutrition. By incorporating the principles outlined in this cookbook, readers can take proactive steps towards improving their symptoms, enhancing their overall health, and reclaiming control over their well-being.

Throughout the cookbook, readers are provided with a wealth of information on PCOS and its dietary implications, including the role of insulin resistance, hormonal balance, and inflammation in the condition. They are guided through practical strategies for creating a PCOS-friendly diet, such as incorporating nutrient-dense foods, balancing macronutrients, and managing portion sizes.

The cookbook offers a diverse range of delicious and nutritious recipes tailored specifically for individuals with PCOS. From indulgent desserts made with PCOS-friendly ingredients to flavorful smoothies packed with nutrients, readers are empowered to enjoy a wide variety of satisfying meals while supporting their health goals.

Furthermore, the cookbook emphasizes the importance of lifestyle factors such as regular exercise, stress reduction, and adequate sleep in conjunction with dietary changes for optimal PCOS management. By adopting a holistic approach to health and wellness, readers can address the multifaceted nature of PCOS and cultivate sustainable habits for long-term success.

Overall, the "PCOS Diet Cookbook for Beginners" equips readers with the knowledge, tools, and recipes needed to navigate their journey towards better health and well-being with confidence and empowerment. Whether you're just starting out on your PCOS management journey or looking for fresh inspiration in the kitchen, this cookbook serves as a valuable resource for anyone seeking to thrive despite the challenges of PCOS.

Thank you for exploring our PCOS Diet Cookbook. Your decision to prioritize your health and well-being by seeking out resources like this demonstrates your commitment to managing Polycystic Ovary Syndrome (PCOS) with diligence and determination.

We understand that navigating the complexities of PCOS can be overwhelming, but we believe that knowledge is power. By arming yourself with the information and recipes contained within this cookbook, you are taking proactive steps towards reclaiming control over your health and embracing a lifestyle that supports your unique needs.

We are grateful for the opportunity to be a part of your journey towards better health and wellness. Our hope is that the recipes and guidance provided in this cookbook will inspire you to discover new flavors, nourish your body with wholesome ingredients, and cultivate habits that promote balance and vitality.

Remember, you are not alone in this journey. There is a community of individuals with PCOS who are facing similar challenges and triumphs every day. Together, we can support and empower each other to thrive despite the obstacles we may encounter.

Once again, thank you for choosing our PCOS Diet Cookbook. We commend you for your dedication to self-care and wish you continued success on your path towards optimal health and well-being.